*Designing Digital Experiences for
Positive Youth Development*

Designing Digital Experiences for Positive Youth Development

From Playpen to Playground

Marina Umaschi Bers

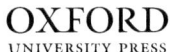

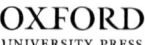
UNIVERSITY PRESS

Oxford University Press, Inc., publishes works that further
Oxford University's objective of excellence
in research, scholarship, and education.

Oxford New York
Auckland Cape Town Dar es Salaam Hong Kong Karachi
Kuala Lumpur Madrid Melbourne Mexico City Nairobi
New Delhi Shanghai Taipei Toronto

With offices in
Argentina Austria Brazil Chile Czech Republic France Greece
Guatemala Hungary Italy Japan Poland Portugal Singapore
South Korea Switzerland Thailand Turkey Ukraine Vietnam

Copyright © 2012 by Oxford University Press, Inc.

Published by Oxford University Press, Inc.
198 Madison Avenue, New York, New York 10016
www.oup.com

Oxford is a registered trademark of Oxford University Press

All rights reserved. No part of this publication may be reproduced,
stored in a retrieval system, or transmitted, in any form or by any means,
electronic, mechanical, photocopying, recording, or otherwise,
without the prior permission of Oxford University Press.

Bers, Marina Umaschi.
 Designing digital experiences for positive youth development : from playpen to
playground / Marina Umaschi Bers.
   p. cm.
 ISBN: 9780199757022
 1. Technology and children. 2. Internet and children. 3. Digital media.
4. Youth development. I. Title.
 HQ784.T37B47 2012
   303.48'3083—dc23   2011026865

9 8 7 6 5 4 3 2 1
Printed in the United States of America
on acid-free paper

Para mami . . . con todo el amor que nos cuesta poner en palabras.

CONTENTS

Acknowledgments   ix

Introduction   3

Part I: The Digital Landscapes for Youth
Overview   19
1. Digital Playgrounds vs. Virtual Playpens in Early Childhood   21
2. Multimedia Parks vs. Virtual Malls in the Elementary Years   36
3. Wireless Hangouts vs. A Palace in Time During High School   52
Summary   62

Part II: A Framework for Designing Digital Landscapes for Personal Development
Overview   63
4. Creating Digital Content to Promote Competence   67
5. Creativity to Build Confidence   82
6. Choices of Conduct to Develop Character Traits   91
7. Communication for Promoting Connections   101
8. Collaboration to Form Caring Networks   111
9. Community Building as Contribution   119
Summary   128

Part III: Plotting Learning Trajectories Through Design
Overview   131
10. Programs and Policies   133
11. From Developing Curriculum to Designing Experiences   135
12. Case Studies   140

Conclusion   175
References   178
Index   190

ACKNOWLEDGMENTS

Although I am the single author for this book, I did not write it alone. Many people, over many years, have contributed their thoughts and ideas to slowly help me shape this book. I had wonderful mentors at the MIT Media Lab, Seymour Papert, Mitchel Resnick, Sherry Turkle, and Justine Cassell; and at Buenos Aires University, Anibal Ford (who sadly passed away recently, with too many ideas still to write) and Alejandro Piscitelli. Rabbi Sergio Bergman has been a constant inspiration for my work, a dear mentor, and a wonderful friend for over two and a half decades.

At Tufts University I have many colleagues who have contributed to the formation of these ideas, but I owe most of my learning about positive youth development to Rich Lerner. I also want to thank Chris Rogers, who shares my passion for design and invention; Don Wertlieb and David Henry Feldman for helping me navigate the Tufts culture; and Debbie LeeKeenan and former colleague Becky New for introducing me to early childhood education. All of my colleagues at the Eliot Pearson Department of Child Development believe in interdisciplinary work and applied research and provide an intellectual home for conducting this work.

However, none of my projects can happen without the smart and hard-working students and research assistants in my DevTech research group at Tufts. Many of them have contributed vignettes for this book, and others have helped with editing of the manuscript and discussion of the underlying ideas for this book at different stages of development. A deep thank-you goes to Clement Chau, Laura Beals, Keiko Satoh, Emily Lin, Hera Kan, Elizabeth Kazakoff, Louise Flannery, Amanda Sullivan, Nauman Kahn, Mike Horn, Jordan Crouser, David Kiger, Rachael Fein, Ken Lee, Nehama Libman, Ethan Peritz, Amanda Puerto, Adriana Flores, and Kathryn Cantrell. Working with all of them is one of the aspects I enjoy most in my academic life. I am deeply thankful to Dave Kahle, Matthew McVey, and David Grogan, from Academic Technologies, for their support over the years; to Ziva Mann for reading an early first draft; and to Joel Segel for helping me with the choice of title.

When one's research involves using technology in the real world, and not only in a lab setting, many people are essential to the project's success. I would like to thank the many teachers, principals, and children I have worked with, especially Jared Matas and Ruth Gass at JCDS, Boston's Jewish Community Day School and the wonderful medical researchers Dr. Dave R. DeMaso, Dr. Joe Gonzalez-Heydrich, and Dr. Betsy Bloom and other medical staff at Boston Children's Hospital and Tufts Medical Center. They were first curious, and maybe a little skeptical, about the potential of virtual communities to help sick children, but then they became true collaborators. Their commitment to the well-being of their young patients constantly reminds me of the importance of taking our research outside the academic ivory tower in a sustainable way.

But of course, believing in ideas is not enough; financial support is an important aspect for doing research. I want to thank the National Science Foundation for supporting interdisciplinary research such as mine, as well as the Noonan Medical Foundation and the Tisch College of Citizenship and Public Service at Tufts University.

While money is important, it is not all. Love and emotional support are even more important for giving us the freedom and peace of mind to conduct the research we are truly passionate about. I want to thank my wonderful friends in Boston and my sisters by choice in Buenos Aires, who have shared tears and laughs over the last three decades. I also want to thank my family: my mother, Lydia Umaschi; my brother, Santiago Umaschi; my sister-in-law, Stephanie Sheppard Umaschi; my aunt Betty Groiso; and my cousin Sergio Schmukler. They are always present when I need them the most, and they have all been very close to me during recent difficult times. The memory of my father, Hector Gerardo Umaschi, inspires me to make the world a better place and to never give up on my dreams. But the most important of all the thank-you's, the very big "Muchas gracias," is for my children, Tali, Alan, and Nico. Tali, big smile and always ready to learn new things, inspires me with her kindness and imagination. Alan, deep eyes and always curious about the world, inspires me with his ability to ask difficult questions and his sensitivity. Nico, beautiful laugh and always easygoing, inspires me with his spark and his creativity. Tali, Alan, and Nico . . . this book is for the three of you. Los quiero mucho.

*Designing Digital Experiences for
Positive Youth Development*

Introduction

We are the children of our landscape; it dictates behavior and even thought in the measure to which we are responsive to it.

—Lawrence Durrell

This book is about children, technology, and human development. However, it is also a book about space. Most specifically, this book is about intentionally designed spaces for children to play, learn, and interact. In the process they engage in the developmental tasks that psychologists have described. But we cannot explore the spaces in this book by taking a stroll. These spaces are digital. And we are immersed in them without 3-D glasses or virtual reality.

Think about landscapes. Some landscapes are natural, unaffected by human activity. However, most landscapes are not only impacted but also designed by humans. Think about landscape designers and architects who master the art and science of arranging and modifying space for aesthetic or functional reasons. This book is about designing digital landscapes with a developmental purpose, to support positive outcomes for children and teens. Yes, positive. There is intentionality, value judgment, and a sense of right and wrong regarding the best digital spaces for our children. This book takes a stance. It is driven by values. It is also driven by a sense of urgency—as the design of our digital landscape is increasingly guided by commercial purposes and not by developmental concerns.

The premise of this book is that understanding our digital landscape as a designed space provides us with opportunities to become landscape designers, as opposed to merely users, consumers, or critics. We don't need to build the technologies ourselves, in the same way that landscape designers don't make the plants or natural resources that they utilize. There is a vast selection on offer, and they can choose what to use, if they learn how to choose. Here, again, is where values come into this discussion.

Landscape designers take into account contextual factors such as soil, drainage, and climate; the survival of plants depends on those. In a similar way, as designers of a digital landscape that promotes positive development, we take into consideration the children's social, emotional, cognitive, physical, civic, and spiritual needs. But we also consider the unique design features of each technology and the practices and policies that shape different interactions in the digital landscape. Like landscape designers, in the 21st century we have a vast array of materials to choose from. But we need a framework to guide our choices. This book provides such a framework: Positive Technological Development (PTD). PTD informs the design of a digital landscape that promotes good, developmentally appropriate experiences with technology.

Although this book is about new technologies, it is inspired by an old question: "How should we live?" The pressing issue is not what kind of digital landscapes we will build, but what kind of people we will become as we inhabit those spaces. This book presents an approach to help children gain the technological literacies of the 21st century while developing a sense of identity, values, and purpose. PTD informs the design of digital spaces so children can use new technologies to become better people and to make the world a better place.

Too often youth's experiences with technology are framed in negative terms (e.g., cyberbullying, sexual predation, invasion of privacy, addiction to video games, etc.). This book acknowledges those problems and risks and takes an interventionist perspective. It invites readers not only to observe and describe the digital landscape but to actively engage in designing it. We want a digital landscape for children and youth to develop as grounded individuals who can contribute to society. This book provides the tools for working toward that goal. No need to be an engineer or a computer scientist to become a partner in crafting our digital landscape.

The book focuses on the developmental span, from preschool to high school, by using landscape design as a metaphor. In the early years, physical spaces are purposefully designed to promote positive development. For example, the carefully designed playground provides a safe space for creative exploration and motor skill development, and the multipurpose park in the elementary school years supports children to find their own interests and develop varied competences and a sense of mastery. As children grow there are few physical spaces purposefully designed to meet their developmental needs. Tweens and teens get together in malls to satisfy their need for social interactions, and they use the Internet, in all of its potential, to engage in their developmental quest. Part I of the book will explore in depth each of these developmental spaces.

But first, let's explore the concept of Positive Technological Development. PTD is a framework that provides an alternative to the deficit discourse about youth's experiences with technology. But most important, it is a tool for all of us to become designers of the digital landscape and make wise choices when working with children and technology throughout the developmental span. In the next section, I will present the PTD framework, and I will briefly introduce the two interdisciplinary theoretical traditions that inspired it: applied developmental sciences and learning sciences. But first, a personal story.

A PERSONAL QUEST

For over a decade and a half, when people asked me what my research was about, I responded: *"Using technology to help children learn new things to become better people and make a better world."* Most people were puzzled. "You mean teaching engineering so children can build bridges in the developing world?" "Are you using new software to increase math scores so children grow to become scientists and can make lifesaving discoveries?" My answer was *maybe*. Although those would certainly be good outcomes, my focus was different. I was helping children, and the adults in their lives, to use new technologies to create projects that they deeply cared about, so they could learn a little bit more about themselves and the personal and cultural values they cherished, so they could explore, in a developmentally appropriate way, three basic questions about being human: "Who are we?" "Where do we come from?" and "Where are we going?" These are the existential questions that, as human beings, we struggle with. At different stages in our lives, we respond to them in different ways, and we find some more challenging than others.

In the process of using technology, children were able to develop an understanding of how computers work, and they were learning powerful ideas from computer programming and applying computational thinking to other aspects of their lives. They were also exploring a varied set of content domains, depending on the chosen project. Some children became experts in dinosaurs so they could build robotic ones with jaws that could open and close. Others knew everything about the flying trapeze so they could engineer its mechanisms with a LEGO™ model. Some learned about ancient cultures, like the Aztecs, so they could create a simulation of their agricultural system, and a few others learned about Hassidic rabbis and Taoist masters so they could program interactive characters to tell inspirational stories about those traditions. Many children built virtual cities and developed their codes of conduct, exploring the challenges of legal systems. Most children worked hard to learn how to program interactive objects, and others learned about organ transplantation so they could make a computer game to teach about organ donation. Over a decade and a half of research, there is amazing breadth and depth in the kinds of computer projects that children did. However, these children were doing something else than developing technological skills. They made connections, formed communities, explored their heritage, helped each other, and took confident steps into academic disciplines of their choice.

At the time, I did not have succinct words to describe my approach to working with children and new technologies. I was simply "using technology to help children learn new things to become better people and make a better world." At first sight, all the pilot projects seemed different. Some were at schools; others, in after-school settings; a few, in museums; and many, in children's hospitals. Some projects engaged four and five year olds, many preteens and teens, and other children in elementary school. Over the years I have used the same approach with a developmentally appropriate focus. The technologies I have designed and used are very different—robotic tools, virtual worlds, storytelling environments, and programming languages.

However, there is a "pattern that connects," as Gregory Bateson put it when he wrote about the "pattern which connects the orchid to the primrose and the dolphin to the whale and all four to me" (1972). The connectedness was in my goal of "using technology to help children learn new things to become better people and make a better world." But at the time, I needed a more sophisticated way to express it. Being an academic, and not an activist, I needed to develop a theoretical framework and conduct empirical studies to validate it. That is the beginning of the story of how the Positive Technological Development framework was born.

During my doctoral studies at the MIT Media Lab working with Seymour Papert and Mitchel Resnick, I was inspired by Constructionism, an approach that could help me address the first part of my stated goal: "using technology to help children learn new things." Constructionism, and its focus on tools for helping children learn by doing, making, and programming, provided me with the intellectual and technological tools to tackle this challenge. However, this theoretical tradition lacked insight into the second part of the sentence, "to become better people and make a better world." Years later, when I joined the faculty of the Eliot Pearson Department of Child Development at Tufts University I learned about applied developmental psychology and, most specifically, about positive youth development. I was then able to find a theoretical framework for the second part of the sentence that summarizes my goal. Over the years, I coined a new term, *Positive Technological Development*. PTD is inspired by and integrates both theoretical traditions. The concept of PTD offers a lens to explain my own approach for "using technology to help children learn new things to become better people and make a better world."

THE NEED FOR POSITIVE TECHNOLOGICAL DEVELOPMENT

To understand PTD as a framework, we first need to learn how the idea of using computers for teaching and learning came about. Based on their pedagogical goals and the design features of the software and hardware, Timothy Koschman (1996) categorizes educational technologies in four groups: computer-assisted instruction (CAI), intelligent tutoring systems (ITS), constructionist authoring environments, and tools for computer-supported collaborative learning (CSCL). While all technological learning environments developed within these four paradigms have the goal to enhance children's cognitive development, they differ in their theoretical stance on *how* to reach that goal.

Borrowing from behaviorism, CAI takes a drill and practice approach. As examples, we can look at software packages that teach numbers and vocabulary by presenting children with simple exercises that are repeated over and over. Later on, with the early developments of cognitivism and artificial intelligence, intelligent tutoring systems started to emerge. Software was designed to iteratively adapt its computerized educational curriculum to match the ability of the student users. Both CAI and ITS systems were developed as stand-alone learning materials that may or may not require supervision from teachers or adults. The content was produced by the designer of the educational software, and the role of the children was to learn it.

In parallel to this growing trend in educational software, a new paradigm emerged: Constructionism. The focus shifted. The child became a producer, rather than a consumer of content. Constructionism advocated for technological tools that support children to become designers and creators of their own personally meaningful computer-based projects. For example, the Logo programming language allowed children to give commands to a turtle to draw on the screen (Papert, 1980). Constructionist tools are often open-ended and require that children learn how to program. While engaging with them, children develop computational literacy and technological fluency and learn to reflect on their own thinking and learning. As a strong inspiration for PTD, Constructionism will be described in depth in the next section.

With the development and growth of the Internet, a new paradigm emerged: computer-supported collaborative learning. The educational tools developed within the CSCL approach involve communication and collaboration among students and among students, parents, and teachers. The focus shifted from an individual student learning with the computer to communities of learners working together to build knowledge via the computer. Strongly grounded in the interdisciplinary field of the learning sciences, CSCL brought community aspects to Constructionism but did not always incorporate the constructionist mandate of learning by making and thinking by programming. However, both paradigms advocated the importance of developing computer literacy and technological fluency.

From an outsider's perspective, both terms—*computer literacy* and *technological fluency*—are similar. Both address what it means to successfully use technology for teaching and learning (Committee on Information Technology Literacy, 1999). However, there is a difference between these constructs. Computer literacy, defined by researchers such as Luehrmann (1981, 2002), Hoffman and Blake (2003), and Livingstone (2004), is about developing instrumental skills to improve learning, productivity, and performance by mastering specific software applications for well-defined tasks, such as word processing and e-mail, and knowing the basic principles of how a computer works. Instead, the construct of technological fluency, first coined by Seymour Papert (1980) and researchers working within the constructionist paradigm, also involves mastering instrumental skills but focuses on enabling individuals to express themselves creatively with technology.

The concept of technological *fluency* (in contrast to mere *literacy*) makes use of the word *fluency* as the ability to use and apply technology as effortlessly and smoothly as people use language. For example, a technologically fluent person can use technology to write a story, make a drawing, model a complex simulation, or program a robotic creature (Papert & Resnick, 1995). As with learning a second language, fluency takes time to achieve and requires hard work and motivation.

To express ourselves through a poem, we first need to learn the alphabet. In the same spirit, to create a digital picture or program a robot, we first need to learn how to use the keyboard and navigate the interface. Thus we need computer literacy. However, although skills with specific applications are necessary, they are not sufficient for individuals to prosper in the Information Age, when new practices and dispositions are constantly needed because applications change rapidly and emerging tools require new skills.

While learning the alphabet is required to write a poem, it is not enough. In the same spirit, knowing how to use software packages is not enough to become technologically fluent. As suggested by the Committee on Information Technology Literacy in 1999, the *"skills" approach lacks "staying power."* Computer literacy is a fundamental stepping-stone toward technological fluency. However, this book strongly argues that technological fluency is not enough if our goal is "using technology to help children learn new things to become better people and make a better world."

Young people use computers to communicate with friends, to listen to and exchange music, to meet new people, to share stories with relatives, to organize civic protests, to shop for clothing, to engage in e-mail therapy, and to find romantic partners, among many other things (Buckingham & Willett, 2006; Ito et al., 2009; Subrahmanyam & Greenfield, 2008). While all of these activities might be facilitated by developing computer literacy and technological fluency, the "life skill set" needed goes beyond them. Even more, the ability to use technology meaningfully rests not only on skills but also on a variety of psychosocial, cultural, and emotional factors (Coffin & MacIntyre, 1999).

The Positive Technological Development framework attempts to provide a model for how development can be supported by the use of technologies. Developing competence and confidence in the use of computers, as the computer literacy and technological fluency movements propose, is important. PTD builds on this work. But it also brings forward the need for youth to develop character traits that will help them use technology safely to communicate and connect with other people and to envision the possibility of making a better world through the use of computers (Bers, 2007b; Ribble, Bailey, & Ross, 2004). PTD is not only about children becoming programmers, engineers, or active in social networks; it is also about helping them find meaning and purpose in life. PTD is in alignment with current Information and Communication Technology Standards, such as the Framework for 21st Century Learning, which emphasize the integration of both technical skills and an understanding of the ethical and social issues surrounding the use of such new technologies (Partnership for 21st Century Skills, 2007).

As a theoretical framework, PTD is a natural extension of the computer literacy and the technological fluency movements that have influenced the world of education since the 1970s but adds psychosocial, civic, and ethical components to the cognitive ones (Bers, 2008a, 2010b). The focus is on positive process: what are children already doing *well* with the technology? PTD builds on the tradition of positive youth development (Benson, Scales, Hamilton, & Sesma, 2006; Damon, 2004), which looks at pathways of thriving individuals in the first two decades of their lives. The underlying assumption is that youth are already using technologies in many positive ways. Our job is to design digital spaces so they can use them in better ways, not only to socialize or learn new things but also to construct a strong sense of identity and promote positive changes in their own selves and society. Our digital landscapes must support children in exploring the developmental milestones for healthy and productive psychosocial growth at each stage.

PTD takes an interdisciplinary approach that integrates ideas from the fields of computer-mediated communication, computer-supported collaborative learning, and constructionist learning with technology, with research in applied developmental science and positive youth development. PTD examines the developmental tasks of a child growing up in our digital era and provides a model for developing and evaluating technology-rich youth programs. The explicit end goal of PTD programs is to mentor children in the positive uses of technology to lead more fulfilling lives—not only to teach children to use technology to accomplish a task, such as the computer literacy movement would have claimed, or solely to help them to design and program their own meaningfully interactive projects, like those who seek technological fluency.

THEORETICAL MODEL

The Positive Technological Development framework involves three components: individual assets, technology-mediated behaviors or activities, and applied practice. The use of the term *positive* connotes the goal of engaging a young person in a good, healthy, and productive developmental trajectory (i.e., development toward improvement of one's self and society).

Individual assets are useful and valuable qualities of a child that provide an advantage or resource for achieving positive outcomes. The Search Institute defines developmental assets as "the relationships, opportunities, and personal qualities that young people need to avoid risks and to thrive." Lerner et al. (2005) frame the various developmental assets into a model of six "C's," conceived as pathways to promote thriving and healthy communities: competence (cognitive abilities and behavioral dispositions), connection (positive bonds with people and institutions), character (integrity and moral centeredness), confidence (positive self-regard, a sense of self-efficacy), caring (human values, empathy, and a sense of social justice), and contribution (orientation to contribute to civil society). The PTD framework extends these assets to the technological domain. Thus, the individual assets or six C's presented are

- **Competence**. An ability to use technology, to create or design projects to accomplish a goal, and to debug projects and problem-solve.
- **Confidence**. A sense of oneself as someone who can act and learn to act successfully in a technology-rich environment, find help when necessary, and have perseverance over technical difficulty.
- **Character**. A moral compass that guides the use of technology in responsible and safe ways and the ability to express one's values using technology.
- **Caring**. A sense of compassion and willingness to respond to the needs and concerns of other individuals, to assist others with technical difficulties, and to use technology as a means to help others.
- **Connection**. Positive bonds and relationships established and maintained by the use of technology.
- **Contribution**. An orientation to contribute to society by using and proposing technologies to solve community/social problems.

The first three C's (competence, confidence, and character) get into the intrapersonal domain, while the other three assets (caring, connection, and contribution) are about the interpersonal domain and refer to individuals as members of a community. Both intrapersonal and interpersonal assets can be expressed, developed, and promoted through the use of new technologies. Technologies provide a platform for people to engage in different activities and behaviors in response to the available design features of the technologies. For example, if the technology provides a writing tool, the user will be able to write a poem or a letter. This is obvious, but it is a key conceptual element to keep in mind, particularly as the desired behaviors supported by the technologies become more complex.

The PTD activities that might lead to positive outcomes for children are presented as a second set of C's that refer to technology-mediated behaviors. These are

- **Content creation**. The opportunity to engage users in computer programming or computer applications that engage them in working with text, video, audio, graphics, and animations. In the process of creating content, children also develop technological fluency. There is a strong relationship between content creation and competence. A sense of *competence* in the technological domain is displayed by the ability to

use diverse computer applications to *create content*, to debug projects, and to problem-solve.
- **Creativity**. The ability to transcend traditional ideas, rules, patterns, relationships, or interpretations and to create and imagine original new ideas, forms, and methods for using new technologies. Most constructionist tools that support content creation also support creativity. There is a strong relationship between creativity and a sense of *confidence*, which is further promoted when one can use technology in *creative ways*.
- **Choices of conduct**. The opportunity of making choices about our behaviors, explore "what if" situations, take action in the digital world, and experience its consequences. There is a relationship between choices of conduct and character. The moral compass that guides the use of technology in responsible ways is built upon having *choices of conduct* and the freedom to evaluate consequences of different "what if" situations and develop a sense of *character*.
- **Communication**. The process of interchanging thoughts, opinions, or information by using technologies. When the mechanisms for supporting *communication* are established, it is possible to envision ways of using technology to *connect* with others. New developments in social media promote new ways of communication.
- **Collaboration**. The opportunity to work with others and to willingly cooperate toward a shared task. There is a strong bidirectional relationship between *collaboration* and *caring*. In order to collaborate we need to care about each other's ideas and needs. The more we establish and maintain positive bonds and relationships, the more we are also able to better collaborate. Most technologies that support collaboration also provide ways for people to connect and communicate.
- **Community building**. An active stance toward using technology to enhance the community and the quality of relationships among the people of that community. Engaging in *community building* has a strong relationship with an orientation to *contribute* to society by using and inventing new digital tools to solve social problems.

The above paragraphs present two different sets of six C's. The first focuses on both intrapersonal and interpersonal assets that can be developed through the use of technology. The second set refers to behaviors that users can engage in through the design affordances of the technologies. However, both our potential for engaging in a developmental and learning process that can promote individual assets and the potential of the design features of the technologies to support certain kinds of

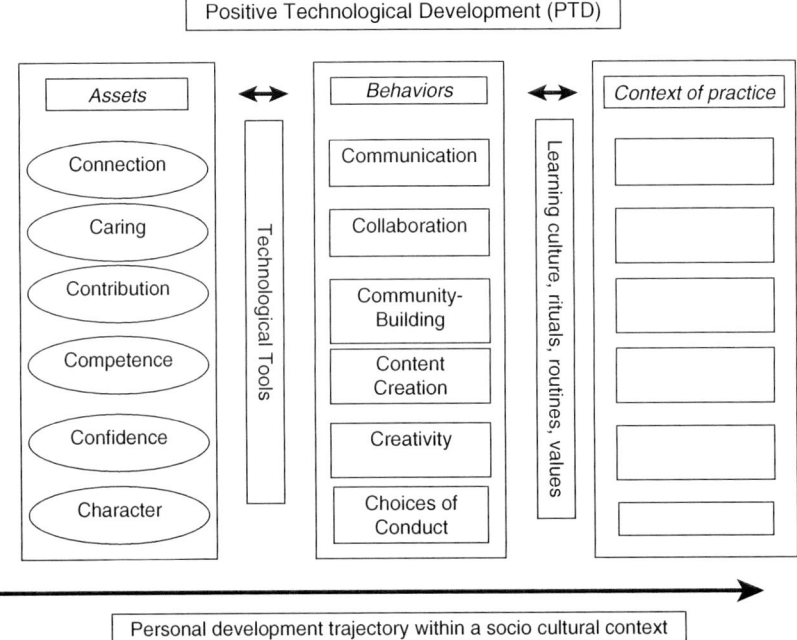

Figure I.1. The Positive Technological Development framework.

activities are mediated by the context in which those technologies are used—the learning culture, rituals, routines, values, or "ways of doing things." Thus, the third element of the PTD framework is the concept of situated practice. It can be a classroom, a hospital, a museum, or the open field of the digital landscape. Figure I.1 summarizes all of these but leaves blank the boxes for the Context of Practice, as it cannot be prescribed for all but, rather, should be specific to each particular context. As the book progresses, I will provide different examples from my various research projects.

This section provided a first introduction to the PTD framework. Part II of the book will revisit it in more depth by focusing on each of the pairs of C's and by providing specific contexts of practice. But before that, we will explore the two bodies of work that have inspired the PTD approach. The first one, Constructionism, developed by Seymour Papert, a pioneer in the field of educational technologies, focuses on children's learning through and about computers. The second one, positive youth development, grew out of research in applied developmental science and pays attention to the overall development of young people as positive contributors to their own growth and society.

CONSTRUCTIONISM: LEARNING BY MAKING, THINKING BY PROGRAMMING

> It would be particularly oxymoronic to convey the idea of constructionism through a definition since, after all, constructionism boils down to demanding that everything be understood by being constructed.
>
> —Seymour Papert

Constructionism is a theory of learning with and about computers developed by Seymour Papert in the late 1970s (Papert, 1980). Papert, a mathematician, an expert in artificial intelligence, and a collaborator of Jean Piaget, pioneered the idea that computers could become wonderful tools for helping children learn new things and think in new ways. At the time, given that computers were big expensive machines that required advanced mathematical skills, it wasn't so clear that Papert's vision would one day be realized. However, in 1967, based at the MIT Artificial Intelligence Lab, he led the team that developed Logo, the first programming language to immerse children in the joy of math land. Logo, a child-friendly version of the programming language Lisp, allowed children to manipulate a turtle on the computer screen to follow their instructions and draw geometrical shapes. In the process, they explored in a fun way concepts of geometry, variables, and recursion while thinking about their own approaches and strategies for learning.

The widespread use of Logo began with the advancement of personal computers during the late 1970s. Papert's ideas became widespread in the world of education in 1980 with the publication of his pioneering book *Mindstorms: Children, Computers, and Powerful Ideas*. Since then, many different versions of Logo have developed. It has been translated into several languages and is widely used all over the world. Logo initiated an era in which Piaget's constructivist theories were applied to understand how children could best use computers to learn. To remind readers about the Piagetian roots of his philosophy, Papert coined the term *Constructionism*, replacing *constructivism*. He wanted to stress the importance of constructions in the world, most specifically on the computer screen, to support the construction of knowledge in our heads. Constructionism states that children learn better when making their own projects, constructing their own ideas, and designing their own solutions to problems. It shows that computers are powerful tools to support and augment all of those activities by providing tools for children to playfully design their own "objects to think with" (Bers, 2008a, 2008b; Kafai & Resnick, 1996).

Following on the Logo tradition, Constructionism asserts the need of authoring systems and programming environments, both software and hardware, to invite children to become designers and programmers of personally and epistemologically meaningful projects (Resnick, Martin, Sargent, & Silverman, 1996). While Logo grew from Papert's love of mathematics, other constructionist programming systems engage children in learning about complex systems (Resnick, 1994), encourage peer learning and collaboration in virtual communities (Bruckman, 1998), promote storytelling skills and the exploration of cultural identity and moral values (Bers, 1998, 2001), and engage children in engineering by making their own robots (Bers, 2008a, 2010a; Bers, Ponte, Juelich, Viera, & Schenker, 2002; Martin, Mikhak, Resnick, Silverman, & Berg, 2000; Resnick, et al., 1996; Rogers & Portsmore, 2004).

Most recently, the Scratch programming environment was developed by Mitchel Resnick and his Lifelong Kindergarten group at the MIT Media Lab. Scratch makes it easy to create interactive stories, games, and simulations by snapping together digital programming elements or blocks, as one would snap together LEGO bricks or puzzle pieces. These projects can then be shared with an active worldwide online community. In the process of creating and sharing projects, young people learn core computational concepts while also learning important strategies for designing, problem solving, and collaborating (Brennan, Monroy-Hernandez, & Resnick, 2010; Resnick et al., 2009).

All constructionist programming environments, from Logo to Scratch, are explicitly designed to situate children in the role of creators of interactive content, as opposed to consumers of information. They all engage children in learning by playing, by exploring, by discovering. And they all encourage children to engage in reflection and to think about their own thinking. Constructionism understands the programming of a computer as a powerful way to gain new insights into how the mind works and learns (Papert, 1993). And most important, it envisions new technologies as powerful carriers of new ideas and as agents of educational change.

Constructionism informs PTD by bringing to the foreground the C's of content creation and creativity and their strong relationship to competence and confidence. The next section will introduce the second body of theoretical work that inspired the PTD framework, positive youth development.

POSITIVE YOUTH DEVELOPMENT: EMPHASIZING STRENGTHS AND ASSETS

> If all teens are thought of as assets in the making, rather than problems waiting to happen, then not only our own families but also society as a whole could be transformed.
>
> —Richard Lerner (2007, p. 213)

Childhood is a relatively new concept. Philippe Aries (1960), by studying the works of art of the medieval period, shows how in those early paintings there are no children, only babies, big adults, and little adults—whom we would call children today. The musculature, dress, expressions, body proportions, and mannerisms are all adult, but in small size. In the medieval world a seven year old was already an adult who would become a worker in the field—or factories during the Industrial Revolution. Aries illuminates how the concept of childhood, as we understand it today, did not always exist in history. It slowly grew into existence in the upper classes in the 16th and 17th centuries, solidified itself in the 18th-century upper classes, and was accepted in the 20th century.

Once the idea of childhood began to develop as a unique life stage, it solidified by taking both an idealist and a deficit model. Children were positioned either as fragile beings who needed to be safeguarded and reformed (Aries, 1960) or as sinful beings whose will had to be broken by flogging and denial (Stone, 1977). Interest in the concept of children as developing individuals began early in the 20th century and started by focusing on abnormal behavior.

Richard Lerner (2007), among other researchers, has shown how in the field of adolescent development, this negative view has influenced decades of research and millions of dollars invested in programs aimed at fixing and preventing problems. Instead of looking at the positive potential, the focus has gone toward the negative possibilities. For example, the term *adolescent* shows this implicit deficit model. In Spanish, my native tongue, it becomes clear. *Adolecer* means "to suffer." By extension, an adolescent is the one who suffers, the one who needs to be helped, the one who is in trouble.

However, in the last decade a new movement started to emerge that focuses on what teenagers are doing right, how they are striving, how they are contributing to society. Using the umbrella term *positive youth development* (PYD), a group of applied developmental scientists started to identify factors that describe teenagers who are not at risk, but, rather, are doing well in life, and to agree on positive characteristics that all young people should possess. Researchers in developmental science (e.g., Damon, 2004; King & Furrow, 2004; Larson, 2000; Scales, Benson, & Mannes, 2006; Theokas & Lerner, 2006) contrast the positive youth development movement as fostering and engendering healthy behaviors with the prevention model that targets at-risk youth before these behaviors even appear.

In his book *The Good Teen*, Richard Lerner (2007) proposes a call for action:

We should think—as a society and as parents—about how to promote healthy, positive, admirable, and productive behaviors in our young people. And we need to find new vocabulary to talk about our young people. Let's name the good things they can and should do. Let's measure these good things. Let's then find ways to make those good things more likely to be present in their lives.

(p. 10)

Above, I described how researchers in the area of PYD use six C's to refer to these developmental assets: competence (cognitive abilities and behavioral dispositions for being healthy), connection (positive bonds with people and institutions), character (integrity and moral centeredness), confidence (positive self-regard, a sense of self-efficacy), caring (human values, empathy, and a sense of social justice), and contribution (orientation to contribute to civil society [Lerner 2002; Lerner & Barton, 2000; Lerner et al., 2005]). Taken together, these characteristics reflect a growing consensus about what is involved in healthy and positive development among people in the first two decades of their lives and the promotion of healthy communities (Scales, Benson, Leffert, & Blyth, 2000).

Research on positive youth development looks at cognitive, personal, social, emotional, spiritual, moral, and civic characteristics of young people in an integrated way. The goal is to understand what goes right in the lives of young people and what could be even better (Lerner, Wertlieb, & Jacobs, 2003). The use of the term *positive* reinforces PYD's emphasis on the promotion of valued characteristics (i.e., developmental assets) that might lead a young person toward a good developmental trajectory (i.e., development toward improvement of one's self and society).

This positive approach provides a framework for implementing and evaluating psychoeducational programs and policies that emphasize the strengths and assets of young people, instead of focusing on diminishing or preventing risk-taking behaviors (e.g., Damon, 2004; King & Furrow, 2004; Larson, 2000; Scales et al., 2006; Theokas & Lerner, 2006). However, most of the youth programs conceived within this model have not attended to the role of new technologies in young people's lives or have limited their use for information delivery or retrieval (Bers, 2006). They have not considered the positive potential of our digital landscape. This omission is particularly striking given that, in today's world, new technologies play an important role in different domains of youngsters lives, such as education, entertainment, socialization, and communication.

The PTD framework hopes to bridge this gap. As shown earlier, it borrows the six C's of PYD and makes them relevant to our digital world. However, instead of only emphasizing developmental assets, it also focuses on behaviors. Technologies are tools that empower individuals to do things, to engage in activities, to act. Therefore, PTD adds a second set of C's focusing on positive behaviors supported by the technology. Our actions in the world change who we are, and who we are changes our actions in the world. There is a bidirectional relationship between developmental assets and technology-supported behaviors. These are mediated by the context provided by the culture, rituals, and values of the environment. The use of technology to achieve certain goals, to act in the world, to make things, doesn't happen in a vacuum but, rather, within a particular sociocultural micro- and macrocultural context.

The goal of PTD is to make the best use of technologies to support children in becoming active agents in their own development and in contributing to society. PTD is both a theoretical framework and a proposed pathway for promoting the best uses of technologies for children and youth in different contexts. Anywhere we can find a digital landscape, PTD might be useful. The next section of the book takes a developmental perspective to visit these digital landscapes.

PART I

The Digital Landscapes for Youth

OVERVIEW

This first part of the book looks at the question of what children and adolescents are currently doing with new technologies and how this is having an impact on their development. It is made up of three chapters that take on a developmental span of children's relationship with technology: early childhood, the elementary years, and high school. Leveraging the concept of landscape, or a space purposefully designed with a goal, each chapter has a central metaphor to illuminate the role of new technologies for promoting the core developmental milestones of each age group. The goal of these metaphors is to help the reader understand the digital world as a developmental space. The hope is to show possible ways for adults to become design partners in its creation. Each chapter is interspersed with vignettes describing children's personal experiences with technology. Some come from my own research projects over the last 16 years. Others come from observing young people's interactions with popular technologies. A summary at the end highlights key ideas visited in this first part of the book.

CHAPTER 1

Digital Playgrounds vs. Virtual Playpens in Early Childhood

Think about a two year old. She is ready to explore the world. She is fearless. She is curious. Everything she finds, she touches, she opens, she closes, she sorts, she hides, she moves, she pushes. She plays. Everyone she encounters, she tries to communicate, she pretends, she asks, she tells, she shows, she gestures. She interacts. Although each child is unique and is influenced by different factors in her environment, research shows that children develop through a generally predictable sequence of steps and milestones. These may not happen in the same way or at the same time for all children, but generally speaking, most two and three year olds enjoy using their senses, their emerging language, and their motor skills to explore the world around them. They can solve simple problems by trial and error. They engage in pretend play by using sticks as swords and puppets as babies. They have a blossoming vocabulary and the ability to understand instructions and situations. They like to play alongside other children, but they do not yet have the capabilities to problem solve in social situations and manage their emotions. This is the age of the "terrible two's," a time in which a child learns how to say no to assert her own sense of self but doesn't yet have the flexibility to take into consideration other people's perspectives or to be aware of her own tiredness.

The American developmental psychologist and psychoanalyst Erik Erikson would describe a two- to three-year-old child as engaging in the developmental task of mastering the physical environment while maintaining self-esteem. Erikson, who was born in Germany in 1902, pioneered the study of the process of identity formation in healthy personalities. Instead of looking at pathologies, he focused on the growth and crises of identity during the different stages of the life cycle. He postulated that every human being goes through eight stages to reach his or her full development, from birth to death. Each of these stages of psychosocial development is marked by a conflict. When there is a successful conflict resolution, there will be a favorable outcome or virtue. The conflict in the preschool years is centered on developing a sense of *autonomy* while avoiding *shame* and *doubt*. When a child can successfully explore this tension, the resulting positive outcome or virtue is willpower, or volition, the process by which an individual decides on and commits to a particular course of action.

For example, a child who learns how to dig a big hole in the backyard on a primary spot next to the flower bed that gave so much work to Mom is very proud of her autonomy to do it by herself. She was able to choose a highly visible and much appreciated place in the yard, to find the right tools and use them effectively, and to carry a project from initial idea to finished product. However, when Mom shows her anger for ruining the flower bed, instead of her praise for the task accomplished, shame and doubt about her own abilities take over this child. She becomes vulnerable. This is an example of the tension that Erikson describes as *autonomy* vs. *shame* and *doubt*. As children grow and enter into kindergarten, this tension intensifies, and Erikson's theory talks about *initiative vs. guilt*, with the resulting virtue as purpose and a sense of accomplishment for intentionally doing an act. For the purpose of this book, I have decided to bring these two stages together and talk about early childhood as a time that extends from preschool into kindergarten. This is a time when playing is an important aspect of healthy child development. As we will see later on, one of the many positive things that technology can do is to support, facilitate, and augment play. As Erikson (2000) writes, "Play is to the child what thinking, planning, and blueprinting are to the adult" (p. 195).

Playgrounds are one of the most popular spaces where young children play. Playgrounds are specifically designed to support the exploration of the physical environment and the development of motor skills, as well as social interactions. They are also probably one of the few spaces where children of this age can be autonomous. They can go on the slide. They can climb up a structure. Next, they can move to the sandbox and build a castle with another child, and when they get bored, they can run around and ask Dad to push them on the swing. Playgrounds offer a space with controlled autonomy. Parents can sit on the benches and carefully observe what is going on while engaging in conversation with other adults. They don't worry about children running out of sight, as most urban playgrounds are surrounded by a fence. Playgrounds are generally safe, but, as with any space that encourages physical activity and social exchanges, there are some risks involved. A child can fall off the slide, can bump her head on the structure, and can get into a fight in the sandbox. All of these events can drive her to shame and doubt about her own skills. However, if risks did not exist, the child wouldn't develop in a healthy and positive way and wouldn't be ready to move to the next developmental stage.

Now, think of a playpen. These pieces of furniture, big or small, made out of rubber and mesh, wood or plastic, serve to corral children into a safe confined space. Playpens and play yards are in sharp contrast with playgrounds. They are risk-free, as long as they are used within their constraints and children do not try to climb out of them. However, there is no room for autonomous exploration. Children can play with the limited toys that Mom or Dad has decided to put inside the playpen. There is no room for imaginative play. Of course, a playpen that is used for half an hour so Mom can prepare dinner is not harming the child in any way. We are focusing here on the playpen as a metaphor that conveys lack of freedom to experiment, lack of autonomy for exploration, lack of creative opportunities, and lack of risks. And I am opposing this metaphor to the one of the playground, where we can find all of these fundamental activities for growing up. The playground promotes, while the playpen hinders, a sense of mastery, creativity, self-confidence, and open exploration.

As a reader who is interested in the role of technology in children's lives, you might be asking yourself why we are talking about playgrounds and playpens. I am responding with a bold claim. From a developmental perspective, most of today's technologies for young children are playpens and not playgrounds. The most obvious thought is that computer games, like playpens, deprive children of physical activity. But the metaphor goes further than that. Most computer games are marketed as educational because young children can develop pre-academic dispositions and learn about shapes, colors, letters, sounds, and numbers. However, from a developmental perspective, those are not the most important milestones for children in this age range. This is a time for free exploration, for testing boundaries, for socializing, for taking risks in a safe way, for engaging in pretend play, for solving problems, for engaging in creative acts that can display children's autonomy.

If we consider the developmental tasks of a two year old, there is no need to buy software marketed as educational for this age range. This software usually limits the types of interactions that children can have with it. Most software provides tasks with right and wrong answers and thus don't encourage problem solving and logical thinking or exploration and creativity.

From a developmental perspective, this kind of interaction in a technological space is more similar to what happens in a confined playpen than to what happens on an open playground. Although the graphics and the cartoon characters of many edutainment software products are appealing, in terms of developmental value, the child can benefit as much by using open-ended, grown-up software. The challenge of navigating the computer screen provides children with an opportunity to make autonomous choices. For example, playing with a word processor allows children to observe a direct link between cause and effect, such as typing letters and seeing them displayed on the screen or changing their color, size, and shape. But using grown-up software, such as a word processor or a paint program, requires parental assistance and supervision—just like on the playground. Instead, edutainment software can be used like a playpen, and parents can leave their children unsupervised. But there might not be a lot of value added from a developmental perspective.

Don't take me wrong. I do not see any harm in having young children play with "edutainment" for half an hour, as I do not see any harm in having them stay in a playpen while dinner is being prepared. However, if we want to know the impact of children playing with these kinds of computer games, we need to ask questions such as, What kinds of developmental tasks are accomplished through the interactions promoted in this digital landscape? Are children given opportunities to explore and experiment, interact and create, in an autonomous way without following prescribed play patterns restricted by the design of the toys adults choose to give them?

For example, on a playground, although the play patterns dictated by the slide are clear—you should climb up the ladder, sit down, and then slide all the way down—children are able to come up with their own creative uses. They can walk up the slide, they can slide facedown, they can slide with others in a train, and so on. Most important, when children get bored, they are free to move on to the next structure or activity and use their imagination in many different ways. They can control the pace of their choices; they can choose what to do, how, when, and with whom.

Developmentally, this might be similar to the kinds of interactions that young children can have with software such as Kid Pix. This multimedia drawing program allows children not only to create their own artwork but also to animate it and display it as a slideshow. Imagination and open exploration drive the types of interactions that happen in this digital space. The child is showing autonomy by deciding what to make and how but, at the same time, is not sheltered from failing in her attempts. Kid Pix, like other software along the constructionist lines, provides a safe playground, as children cannot go outside its boundaries but, within them, can explore as much as they want. Other examples, such as JumpStart 3D

Virtual World, blend adventure with education. While the tool offers activities to master skills based on national educational standards in math, reading, and critical thinking, the most interesting activities in this digital space, from a developmental perspective, are those that invite children to design a unique avatar, decorate a house, create artwork to display, nurture virtual pets, or choose their own missions to complete. Of course, in this three-dimensional environment, although the avatar can move around, the child is still sitting in front of the computer screen, although she might benefit from physical activity.

Preschool-age children have the cognitive and fine motor skills required to understand that the movement of their hand triggers the mouse movement on the screen. They can also coordinate dragging and dropping and clicking functions. Thus they can engage with current computer interfaces. So, why the need for software such as the programs mentioned above specifically targeted at young children? We can ask a similar question about playgrounds in suburban areas: Why do we need those artificially crafted spaces if children can play in the woods? I am sure you can think of many reasons, but safety and autonomy probably come at the top of the list. While in the woods young children need to be constantly supervised and helped; on the playground children can run free. Parents and caretakers are there, but they can relax and sit on the benches. Also, there are structures already built for them; there is no need to start from scratch every time. Children can subvert their use of the slide and climbers and still engage in creative activities in the sandbox, but someone has thought about landscaping the space with structures that are developmentally appropriate.

The same is true with software specifically designed for children. For example, although from an interface perspective, a child can use Photoshop and PowerPoint as well as Kid Pix, the level of support needed is very different. It is very likely that preschool-age children cannot read. Thus parents might not want them using grown-up software on their own, as the risk of finding parts of the operating system in the recycling bin is too great. Children need pictures and sounds and big objects that can be easily manipulated on the screen. Constructionist types of software such as Kid Pix provide a fence, very much in the way that the playground provides a fence. Parents don't have to supervise or assist their children's every click. They can give them autonomy and promote free exploration. Children can take risks and learn how to learn.

Virtual playgrounds are on the rise for the preschool crowd. For example, Panwapa (http://www.panwapa.com/) is a virtual floating island that travels the five oceans of the world. The goal is to expose children to other cultures. Launched in December 2007 for a target audience of three to five year olds, it was developed in collaboration between Sesame Workshop and Merrill Lynch. Within the first five months, 50,000 children signed up to the site (Shore, 2008). Since most preschoolers don't know how to read and write, traditional text-based communication mechanisms found in virtual worlds are not feasible. Instead, alternate means of communication are necessary, such as using symbols to convey feelings (e.g., icons representing different facial expressions) or having spoken messages. In the Panwapa world, children can communicate with each other by exchanging *Panwapa Cards* with a pre-scripted simple message chosen by the sender, such as, "We like some of the same things, and some different things!" and "I like your house. Please visit mine!" (Beals & Bers, 2010). The messages can also be played out loud. Panwapa is an example of a virtual playground that supports the child in her developmental quest to take on an autonomous role to express her willpower and sense of accomplishment—the developmental milestones that Erikson identifies for this stage.

While some virtual playgrounds involve software, others are physical. For example, at the Rosengårdskolen in Odense, Denmark, a public primary school that serves around 650 students, high-tech learning is not limited to the classroom. The school features a high-tech playground that is linked via the Internet to other playgrounds like it around the world. The structures in the playground call out to students to play games that focus on teamwork and academic skills while incorporating physical activity and fun into the activities. Some of the games are scored, and students can compete with others around the world. My student Jennifer Iassogna spent a semester at the school and observed the many different games children play:

> There is one game that features a set of buttons built into the ground that students jump on. The buttons have to be jumped on in a certain pattern following a game directed by a screen. Based on time and accuracy, students are awarded points, and they can be scored against other students at their own school or on other continents. When it comes to teamwork, there is another game that is played on a large climbing structure where different buttons light up and as a group, the students need to climb and tap them all. The students really enjoy these features on the playground.

This high-tech playground is an example of the different ways in which innovation is happening in early childhood education. In recent years the demand for kid-friendly laptops has been on the rise. Electronics makers are exploring that life period in which parents might not want their young children playing with their own computers, due to their messy habits nd their underdeveloped motor skills, which might result in missing keyboard keys and scratched screens, but do want to expose them to the digital world. They want a safe playground for their children. This is not the same as a playpen: that is, mess-proof toys that look like computers but do not offer open-ended possibilities in terms of software, only limited gamelike applications.

In 2006, the In-Stat market research firm found that 46% of consumers purchased a high-tech gadget for a child three to five years of age, the highest spending level on behalf of any children's age group. There is in the market a growing trend to sell hardware that engages the child in physical activity. But this doesn't necessarily mean that we are getting closer to the playground metaphor. For example, Fisher-Price's Smart Cycle is a beautifully designed stationary bike. As children pedal they are immersed in different games that teach about upper- and lowercase letters, numbers, and shapes. The goal is to reinforce academic skills in a fun and active way. Although there are motor skills involved, in terms of the developmental tasks that are fundamental at this age, this bike is a playpen. It might be useful to burn some energy on rainy days and to entertain little Johnny when Mom is on the phone, and it can also teach him letters before he encounters them at school, but there is little opportunity for creative exploration in an autonomous way—the fundamental developmental task of a preschooler. However, the good news is that the nature of technology is to constantly change. As innovative hardware is developed, we will see more digital playground experiences that involve the use of both fine and gross motor skills.

For now, robotic kits that enable users to make and program "smart" objects that move around and sense the world around them can serve as playgrounds for young children (Bers, 2008a). Children are physically active while playing with them. They use their little hands to build them and their logical thinking to program them. Although most commercially available robotic kits require the child to sit in front of the computer to program the robot's behaviors, some experimental prototypes are exploring a different approach by using tangible programming. Tangible languages, instead of relying on icons and words on a computer screen, use physical objects to represent computer code. Children can arrange and connect these physical elements to construct programs.

Tangible languages exploit the physical properties of objects, such as size, shape, and materials, to express and enforce programming syntax. The idea of tangible programming was first introduced in the mid-1970s (Perlman, 1976) and was revived nearly two decades later (Suzuki & Kato, 1995). Since then several tangible languages for children have been created in different research labs around the world (e.g., Horn & Jacob, 2007; McNerney, 2004; Smith, 2007; Wyeth & Purchase, 2002). At Tufts we have taken a hybrid approach by developing the Creative Hybrid Environment for Robotic Programming (CHERP) system, which enables young children to transition back and forth between the screen-based language and tangible interlocking wooden blocks. Both the on-screen programs and the wooden blocks use the same icons to represent actions for the robots to perform. This hybrid approach allows children to work with multiple representations (Horn, Crouser, & Bers, 2011). Later on in the book, several vignettes and one case study of young children building and programming robots with CHERP will be presented.

To be consistent with the playground metaphor, robotic kits for children must involve two elements: the possibility of creative open-ended construction in the physical world and the possibility of programming the behaviors of the constructed object to be interactive and respond to stimulus via its sensors. Over the years the LEGO company has developed different robotic kits, and several universities and research labs have also implemented their own robotic prototypes (Martin et al., 2000; Rogers & Portsmore, 2001; Rusk, Resnick, Berg, & Pezalla-Granlund, 2008). However, most of these robotic kits have been developed for children who are seven years old and older. Their use is becoming widespread in high schools and middle and elementary schools.

In my own DevTech research group at Tufts University, with funding from the National Science Foundation, we are experimenting with developmentally appropriate programming languages for early childhood education such as CHERP (Bers, 2010b; Bers & Horn, 2010; Horn et al., 2011). Along with LEGO™ bricks, children can build with recyclable materials such as feathers, pipe cleaners, paper, yarn, string, googly eyes, popsicle sticks, water bottles, tissue boxes, straws, and Velcro. Over the years, four and five year olds have built LEGO towns with robots that stand upright and wave their arms to greet town visitors and ballerinas that can sing and dance. Some have created robotic flowers that grow out of the ground when there is light and plants that spin as people approach. Many children have made soccer players that can kick a ball and cars, trucks, and trains that can race with each other and transport animals to the zoo. The possibilities are unlimited (Bers, 2008a).

In a playground approach to working with young children and robotics, there is playful learning, autonomous decision making (even if as adults we know that they will lead to initial failure), and risk taking. Children engage in social interactions and negotiations while playing to learn and learning to play (Resnick, 2003). The Eriksonian tension of "autonomy vs. shame and doubt" that characterizes this stage of development is played out. When making robots, children become engineers by exploring with gears, levers, motors, sensors, and programming concepts. They also become storytellers as they create characters that can move in response to input from the environment (Bers, 2008a). Children work on the floor, on the table, and on the computer and navigate among those physical spaces. They use their hands, struggle to connect small LEGO pieces, glue fabric onto their projects, and run around to test the speed of their cars (Bers, 2008b). Children are physically busy. In the preschool years, development of motor skills is fundamental for later growing.

While robotics can be used as playgrounds that serve the fundamental developmental needs in early childhood, they can also be a gateway to learn applied mathematical concepts, the scientific method of inquiry, and problem solving (Rogers & Portsmore, 2004). Educational robotic kits have been described as a new generation of learning manipulatives that build on the tradition of Montessori and Fröebel (Bers, 2008a; Resnick, 2007a). Those early "manipulatives" and "gifts" were designed for children to develop a deeper understanding of mathematical concepts such as number, size, and shape (Brosterman, 1997). Today most early childhood settings have Cuisenaire rods, pattern blocks, Digi-Blocks, and other manipulatives carefully designed to help children build and experiment. More recently, "digital manipulatives" have expanded the range of concepts that children can explore. For example, researchers at MIT have embedded computational power into toys such as blocks, beads, and balls, so young children can learn about dynamic processes and "systems concepts," such as feedback and emergence, that were previously considered too advanced for them (Resnick, Berg, & Eisenberg, 2000).

However, although robotics support learning about these new concepts and ideas, this is not a fundamental developmental task for young children. Neither is learning letters and numbers, taught by playpen-style educational software. Robotic kits can be wonderful playgrounds for young children because they encourage problem solving and logical thinking, creativity and love of learning, through playful explorations. Teaching the ABC's, numbers, or computational concepts earlier might be appealing but might not make a difference in the long run. While these are activities that can pave the road for later academic transition, the mastery of new practices and knowledge is the fundamental developmental task for the next stage, the elementary school years. We will explore this in the next section.

First, the following three vignettes showcase examples of young children using technology with a digital playgrounds approach as discussed in this chapter. Playground technologies support children in using their creativity and imagination, discovering and inventing, while making their own projects in a playful way. For example, the children described in the next pages used technology by fostering their imaginative play, from creating digital monsters to making fantastical creatures out of robotics to playing make-believe in the Panwapa virtual world.

Vignette 1
A PLAYFUL TOOL FOR LITTLE FINGERS

By Elizabeth R. Kazakoff

Madeline, 2.5 years old, Boston, Mass.
Madeline is a two and a half year old from Boston, Mass. She is the only child of an elementary school teacher and a computer programmer. Madeline's parents love reading to her and playing with her and her toys. Madeline's favorite toys include blocks and stuffed animals. She only watches one TV show—*Sesame Street*.

About six months ago, Madeline's dad bought an iPad. Madeline's parents had heard about educational apps that could be purchased for the iPad but were nervous about giving a young child an expensive piece of technology. One weekend, however, they decided to download a few apps they had read about online and show Madeline.

The first time they showed Madeline the iPad, she climbed onto her mother's lap and looked curiously at the device. "Bella!" she exclaimed, pointing to the photo on the screen of the family's cat. Madeline look at the screen, seemingly puzzled but still very curious. She then touched the screen, her finger landing on an icon. *Wheels on the Bus*, an interactive book, appeared. Madeline looked, at first startled, but then grew very excited, realizing that her little finger had made something appear! Madeline then began touching different objects on the screen. To her amazement, the objects she touched produced actions and corresponding sounds while playing the classic "Wheels on the Bus" song. She sang along to the song, and as she made the horn honk and wipers swish, she looked up at her mother and giggled.

When the song was over, they played it again and again. Eventually, Madeline handed the iPad back to her mother and requested "more photos." Madeline's mother showed her how to press the button at the bottom of the device and how to swipe her finger across the screen to move back to the initial screen. "Now me!" said Madeline. Madeline then swiped her finger back and forth, moving the screen view until she noticed the camera icon and touched it. "More Bella!" she said as she used her finger to scroll through pictures of the cat. "Mommy! Daddy! Me!!!" she continued to shout as she excitedly scrolled through family photos stored on the iPad.

When she was done scrolling through all the photos, she pushed the round button at the bottom of the iPad to return to the main screen. As she did this, something red caught her eye. "Elmo!" Madeline tapped the Elmo button, and Elmo's Monster Maker appeared. Madeline began touching the "monster" on the screen. With each press of her finger, new eyes appeared. She moved her finger lower, and a new nose appeared; higher, and a hat appeared. She quickly moved her finger back and forth, trying to make a silly monster. With each new combination, she would look up at her mother and giggle.

This first experience with the iPad was not her last. Like many young children, Madeline found the iPad intuitive. Madeline loves playing with her mom and dad, singing "Wheels on the Bus," taking and looking at photos, drawing with the paint application, reading along with her parents to her many stored storybooks, and playing vocabulary games. Her parents have created a special folder for Madeline's photos (mostly of Elmo's monster friends) and favorite children's songs.

Madeline's parents had several discussions about how much time she should be spending with the iPad. She typically uses it for a story or game before bed. Her mom or dad is always there to play along with her. They frequently read and draw, sometimes they dance to the stored music, occasionally they build monsters, and often they discuss the memories associated with the stored photos. In Madeline's home, the iPad is just like any other toy or book, except this one can take on a thousand forms in just one small piece of equipment, perfect for little fingers.

Vignette 2
FANTASY PLAY COMES TO LIFE THROUGH A ROBOT

By Louise Flannery

Katerina, five years old, Cambridge, Mass.
Katerina is a kindergartener who lives with her parents and older brother, Gabe, who is eight. She is never shy with adults; has lots of energy, curiosity, and humor; and loves to experiment and learn about new things. Never bored, she creates numerous drawings and other projects with arts and crafts materials. She also builds with blocks at school and with sand, twigs, and water in her yard. Until last week, however, Katerina had never built with Gabe's LEGOs. She had seen Gabe build towers and cars, but those things didn't interest her. How could she play with him? But now Katerina has an idea, because last week she attended a robotics summer camp specially designed for kindergarteners.

At camp, Katerina and the other children learned how to build and program robots to make a robotic town. The robots were made from LEGO robotic parts, LEGO bricks, and arts and crafts materials. The group brainstormed all sorts of possible robots for a town. Many children thought of vehicles (garbage trucks, cargo ships, and army tanks) or buildings with moving parts, like a drawbridge and a door that opens when you push a button. The camp counselors also helped children think of people who live and work in a town, and Katerina decided to try that out. She found a buddy, Elsa, who was also interested in making a robotic person.

Making the robotic person was challenging for several reasons: the girls needed to make the materials work, and they had to collaborate successfully. As they talked about what to do and tried building their person—a farmer—in different ways, they decided that the farmer would greet anyone who walked by. Katerina wanted it to wave its arms, but the motors kept falling off. Their creation did not look as much like a person as they wanted. What could they do? Elsa felt that the farmer should move in some other way or just sing, but Katerina really wanted to fix the waving arms. Finally, after trying out many ideas and getting advice from one of the camp counselors, Katerina and Elsa's robotic farmer had all the necessary parts connected so it could wave its arms, flash its eyes, and sing whenever it sensed someone passing by.

After they completed building it, the girls programmed instructions for their robotic farmer to do all of these things. After a week of hard work, they were ready to show off this project to their parents during the final day of camp. Though the process of making and debugging their robot and program had not always been easy, when they were done, Katerina was proud of their accomplishments. Feeling confident that she could make other projects if she tried, she wished robot camp would last another week. She also felt happy that she had worked with Elsa; she had made a new friend.

Now, a few days since the end of the robotics camp, Katerina is thinking busily about all the challenges she and Elsa had to solve to make their robotic farmer, and she is imagining other robots she'd like to make. While she doesn't have her own robotics set at home, she has been proactive about joining her brother's LEGO play and building all sorts of creatures with paper, tape, and stickers. She now feels confident to connect with Gabe in LEGO play and in her ability to imagine and make interesting objects. She spends time each afternoon building these creations and giving them fantasy robotic capabilities. Someday, she hopes, she will have her own robotics set at home and make robots really come to life.

Vignette 3
A SAFE ONLINE PLAY SPACE FOR A PRESCHOOLER

By Laura Beals

Emma, four years old, Boston, Mass.
Emma is an only child who is very shy. She takes a while to warm up to new situations and people and makes friends slowly, though she has two best friends from school, Jane and Charlotte. Even though she is shy, Emma really enjoys playing make-believe. At school she loves the dramatic play area of the classroom—her teachers notice that when she is pretending to be someone else, she becomes less shy. At home, she spends hours in her playroom with her play kitchen, her play workbench, and her favorite: her play veterinary kit, with her dog, Sammy, being her preferred "patient."

Both of her parents have technology-based careers, thus Emma has been exposed to computers, smart phones, and other technologies from birth. However, her parents are cautious about what technology she is allowed to use; she had very little exposure to television or computers until she was over two years old. They do feel, however, that in today's world it is important for children to be competent with technology in order to be successful in school, and so they are open to her experiencing technology that they feel is age appropriate and which they can explore with her.

Emma had been requesting to "play on the 'puter," and so her parents began researching options for preschoolers and asking other parents at Emma's preschool what their children were using. Her parents had heard about a virtual world created by Sesame Workshop, called Panwapa (http://www.panwapa.com/), and so they explored the Web site in more detail. Her parents were confident in its educational value and appropriateness for their daughter, as Panwapa was developed by the same experts behind *Sesame Street*, using research-based principles. In addition, they appreciated that the Web site had easy-to-find materials for caregivers to better understand the experience and engage in the program with their child. Also, they thought that the five educational principles of the program—*Awareness of the Wider World, Appreciating Similarities and Valuing Differences, Taking Responsibility for One's Behaviors, Community Participation and Willingness to Take Action,* and *Understanding of and Responsiveness to Economic Disparity*—were ones to which they felt Emma should be exposed. Finally, they thought that the make-believe basis of the world, and the fact that Emma would be able to interact with other kids in a safe manner, would be an ideal play experience for their daughter.

Panwapa, developed in collaboration with Sesame Workshop and Merrill Lynch and intended for children ages four to seven, is based on a metaphor of a virtual floating island that travels the five oceans of the world. As of November 2010, there were over 313,000 Panwapa kids. Panwapa's child-friendly interface and activities allow children to be active participants in becoming members of the community via their own initiative. For example, children are encouraged to create their own characters, flags, and houses as well as gather collections of cards such as World Cards (gathered by visiting new places), Rare Animal Cards (gathered by encountering the animal in its native country), Panwapa Islander Cards, and Panwapa Kids Cards. It is through these activities that the Panwapa developers aim to achieve their overarching purpose:

> Technology is drawing people across the world closer together, creating opportunities, and bringing about change. This interconnectedness is also demanding that children develop greater awareness and skills to navigate and thrive in the world.... We believe that today, more than ever, learning how to be a global citizen is fundamental to a child's healthy development.

Emma needed her mom's help when she first joined Panwapa, as she had to request a user name and select a password. She also had to design her character, her house, and her flag—officially called *Panwapa Kids*, *Panwapa Homes*, and *Panwapa Flags*, respectively—before she could enter the world. A Panwapa Kid can be customized with different body colors, eyes, mouths, hairstyles, shoes, and outfits. The shape, building materials, and surroundings can be chosen for a Panwapa Home. To customize a Panwapa Flag, a user chooses one favorite item from each of six categories: food, animals, sports, musical instruments, activities, and crafts. While children can customize each of these three items, their choices for doing so are limited. This limitation is another reason why Emma's parents felt comfortable allowing her to play in Panwapa—there is no opportunity for her to accidentally "stumble" upon inappropriate content within the Panwapa world.

Emma really enjoyed this part of Panwapa—she thought it was very fun to make her character have blue skin, green eyes, and yellow pigtails and to wear a pink-and-white action hero outfit complete with a pink eye mask. She often returned to this part of Panwapa to change her character's look. When she first started Panwapa, she had difficulty using the computer mouse to control her actions on the screen. However, as she continued using Panwapa, she became much better at controlling the mouse and was proud that she could eventually play in Panwapa all by herself most of the time. She still has to ask for help when the browser freezes or if she accidently clicks outside of Panwapa.

One of Emma's favorite activities in Panwapa is to communicate with other Panwapa children using Panwapa Cards. These cards have the child's Panwapa name, picture, and flag. In addition, the Panwapa Cards have a pre-scripted simple message chosen by the sender, such as, "We like some of the same things, and some different things!" and "I like your house. Please visit mine!" As Emma cannot yet read on her own, she loves clicking on the cards because the message is read out loud for her. Her parents are happy that communication is restricted in this manner; they would not feel comfortable if Emma were able to write messages or receive them from other users. Because of this, they feel comfortable allowing her to play in Panwapa on the house computer, which is located in the kitchen, while they are making dinner in the evenings. Her parents have decided to limit her playing in Panwapa to 20 minutes a day during this time. She is not allowed to use the computer, or Panwapa, without asking permission from a parent, and when she is on the computer, a parent frequently checks on what she is doing.

Emma's second favorite activity in Panwapa is a game called "Hide and Seek With Koko," in which Koko, a Muppet character, hides somewhere on the island, giving the child clues in order to find her. There are many opportunities for play in Panwapa, especially make-believe play. In fact, the entire "island" is make-believe, as reinforced by the cast of Muppet characters. Other games in Panwapa, though not Emma's favorite, are "Panwapa Movie Play-Along," in which children can watch and play along with interactive short videos featuring real children from around the world in order to better understand how other children live in very different economic situations from themselves but have the same basic needs, such as food, water, and shelter; and "Treasure Hunt," in which children can follow a series of clues around the Panwapa world in order to find other Panwapa Kids, allowing them to win special Panwapa Cards.

While playing in Panwapa has not made Emma more comfortable making friends, her parents have noticed that her skills in using the computer independently have improved greatly. They also find that she is showing an interest in geography and asks to read books about other places in the world. They do believe that allowing Emma to engage in make-believe in Panwapa for a little bit everyday exposes her to a new avenue for exploration of her imagination. They will continue to let her play with Panwapa until she indicates that she is interested in a new experience; at that time, they will begin the process of finding another age-appropriate virtual experience for Emma.

CHAPTER 2

Multimedia Parks vs. Virtual Malls in the Elementary Years

Think of a nine year old. She wakes up in the morning and after breakfast goes to school. She spends most of the day learning new things and socializing with peers. During recess, she plays outside. Not only does she explore the space and experiment with the objects she finds, as she did in her preschool years, but she also organizes and participates in games. Those games require her to learn rules and engage in social negotiations. She tries to get better at the games every time she plays. There are winners and losers. She is starting to realize that she needs to work hard to get what she really wants. When she comes back home, she participates in after-school activities: soccer, piano, gymnastics, math club, and so on. She has homework, and she has to study for tests. She is learning how to manage her time. She is also learning how to set her own play dates to spend time with friends.

Although the length of the school day and the after-school activities might be different, most children in the elementary school years spend their time learning how to master new skills—academic, physical, and social. Erikson describes this stage of development as *industry vs. inferiority*. A child is capable of working hard to accomplish new skills—successfully solve a math problem, score a goal in a soccer game, or invite a friend for a play date. But she might also feel that she is not as good as her classmates in some or all of these tasks. She starts to compare herself with others, she notices disparities in abilities to achieve, and feelings of inadequacy and low self-esteem may arise. When the tension is successfully solved, the resulting virtue is a strong sense of competence.

In this chapter I am proposing the park as a space for the development of competencies. Most children in elementary school enjoy going to the park. In contrast with the fenced playgrounds of the preschool years, parks are big spaces that allow children to engage in many different activities. There are the traditional play structures such as swings, slides, and sandboxes, but there are also basketball courts, paved roads for biking or scootering, woods for hiking, and open fields for baseball or soccer. There are tables and benches for doing homework or having a picnic and lots of space to walk around. Although in some cases adults walk or drive children to the park, the interactions with the adult don't matter as much as the interactions with peers. At the park children choose their favorite activities; they develop and master skills and engage socially with peers. From a developmental perspective, parks offer opportunities for gaining competence beyond academic disciplines.

Now think of a mall. We find elementary school children who choose to go to the mall with their friends—particularly those children in the older grades. Parents drop them off at the mall entrance and pick them up two hours later or stay with them. Children walk around the mall and look at shops; they might even try on some clothes and sit for a snack at the food court. They can decide how to spend their money and can choose which stores to go into and which ones to ignore. Children are bombarded with commercial advertising. The mall, beyond exposing children to the fundamentals of capitalism, doesn't offer as many opportunities for building competence and mastery, the fundamental developmental tasks at this age, as the park does. Don't take me wrong. Malls can serve a positive function. One goes to the mall to buy something or to walk protected from inclement weather. However, in this chapter, malls are presented as spaces that might serve a developmental function.

Both parks and malls are metaphors for looking at digital landscapes in the elementary school years. While parks offer opportunities for gaining mastery and competence—the fundamental developmental milestones at this stage—malls don't. Malls are spaces for consumption, as opposed to creation. This metaphor holds when taken to the digital world. While some Web sites, video games, programming languages, and virtual worlds engage children in becoming fluent with technology and learning new skills, others merely expose them to sound, color, and animation, as well as multiple ads. Some technologies invite children to create their own projects and demand an investment of time and effort to learn the needed skills. Whereas others provide quick gratification, by having children consume what others have created.

Mitchel Resnick, from the MIT Media Laboratory, writes about "pianos, not stereos":

> The stereo has many attractions: it is easier to play and it provides immediate access to a wide range of music. But "ease of use" should not be the only criterion.

Playing the piano can be a much richer experience. By learning to play the piano, you can become a creator (not just a consumer) of music, expressing yourself musically in ever-more complex ways. As a result, you can develop a much deeper relationship with (and deeper understanding of) music.

(Resnick, Bruckman, & Martin, 1996, p. 41)

A child who learns how to play the piano is engaging in one of the essential developmental tasks for the elementary school years: mastering new skills. Of course, there is a time and place for listening to good music on a stereo (or an iPod), just as there is a time and place for going shopping at the mall. These are all metaphors that highlight the potential role of the child as a consumer or as a producer.

The "pianos, not stereos" motto conveys the idea of the child as producer. However, it limits the domain of mastery to what those particular objects can offer. A space metaphor, instead, opens up the game. A space can house many objects and invite many interactions, so children can experiment with different domains of mastery. Not all children enjoy or are good at music, and not all can or want to invest the energy and effort needed to skillfully play the piano. The park, instead, offers multiple opportunities. A child can play organized sports on the basketball court or the baseball field. She can freely explore the area and become an expert hiker. She can bike around the paths. She can engage in conversations with peers and work at mastering social skills. She can sit on the benches and do homework. The possibilities are endless. The child can choose a domain and master it. And then, she can move on and try a new domain. The park offers, in the words of Sherry Turkle and Seymour Papert (1992), the possibility for "epistemological pluralism," a diversity of new ideas, new ways of knowing, and new approaches to problem solving.

This book looks at technology as a developmental space, not as an object or tool to accomplish a task. However, not all spaces are the same; nor do they afford similar opportunities for personal growth. The multimedia park metaphor, as opposed to the virtual mall, highlights that technologies in the elementary school years should provide opportunities for playful mastery and competence—the virtues identified by Erikson as essential for this stage of development.

This is aligned with the fundamental principle of Constructionism that we visited in an earlier chapter. Constructionist learning environments provide tools for children to become designers and creators of their own projects. Children become producers, as opposed to consumers of content. They can apply concepts, skills, and strategies to solve authentic problems. This philosophy is shared with approaches such as "learning by designing" (Kolodner, Crismond, Gray, Holbrook, & Puntamhekar, 1998), "knowledge as design" (Perkins, 1986), and "design education" (Ritchie, 1995). In constructionist learning environments children create projects that are, first, personally relevant. Children are invested in making them. They care about them; they are interested in them. Second, the projects are epistemologically relevant. Children learn about a particular domain of knowledge and explore powerful ideas in this area. And third, they are sharable. Children can show them and talk about them with a community.

There is a long tradition of constructionist learning environments focused on exposing children to the domain of computer science. Environments such as Logo and Scratch engage children in learning computer programming, either as an epistemologically relevant domain to master for its own sake or as a way to master other domains of knowledge. For example, a child can learn Logo and master the computational concepts of recursion and variables. But she can also apply those concepts to learn geometry while programming the Logo turtle to make squares of different sizes and colors. A child can animate a character using Scratch and learn about computational control structures but can also use those concepts to create an interactive story with all of the structural components of a well-formed narrative.

Programming environments are spaces. The results of the activities that happen in those spaces are objects—virtual or tangible. Although the constructionist literature hasn't explicitly focused on the developmental milestones that children could achieve in those spaces, the emphasis has always been on mastery and competence. Papert coined the term *technological fluency* (Papert & Resnick, 1995), which refers to the ability to use and apply technology in a fluent way, effortlessly and smoothly, as one does with language. For example, a technologically fluent person can use technology to write a story, make a drawing, model a complex simulation, or program a robotic creature. As with learning a second language, fluency takes time to achieve and requires hard work and motivation. In order to gain technological fluency, one should first master basic skills and achieve technological literacy (Bers, 2008a).

Technological literacy has sometimes come to be known as "computer literacy" and has a long history. It refers to the ability to use computer applications, such as a spreadsheet and a word processor, and to search the Internet for information. The Partnership for 21st Century Skills (http://www.21stcenturyskills.org) describes several skills that children need to learn "to succeed as effective citizens and leaders in the 21st century, such as using digital technology, communication tools and/or networks appropriately to access, manage, integrate, evaluate, and create information in order to function in a knowledge economy" (2007).

However, skills with specific computer applications are necessary but not sufficient for individuals to prosper in the Information Age, when new skills are constantly needed, applications change rapidly, and new tools require new skills.

Programming environments provide a venue to help children develop technological fluency. But other digital spaces might also achieve this goal. For example, some video games and virtual worlds offer opportunities for children to become producers, and not only consumers of digital materials.

In 2010, according to a study of 1,200 households by the Entertainment Software Association (ESA), 67% of American households played video games, 64% of parents believed that games are a positive part of their children's lives, and 48% of parents played video games with their kids at least once per week. The term *video games*, as it is used here, refers to software, supported by any type of computer, console, or mobile or virtual platform that involves interaction with a user interface to generate visual feedback on any display by manipulating an input device, such as a game controller, joystick, keyboard, or mouse.

Games are goal-directed and competitive activities conducted within a framework of agreed rules. This ample definition makes room for different genres of games: ludic games, in which players win by taking action and developing strategies; narrative games, in which players solve conflicts by choosing different paths of action; and simulations, in which players can observe emerging behavior patterns to understand how a particular system functions in different circumstances. Playing games might involve racing, solving puzzles, doing sports, engaging in action and adventure, playing with rhythm and music, developing strategies, participating in simulations, fighting, first-person shooting, or role-playing. As of 2009, the best-selling video games were sport games (19.6%) and action games (19.5%), followed by family entertainment (15.3%) and shooter games (12.2% [ESA, 2010]). The top games sold for families were Super Mario Bros., several Wii games such as Wii Play® and Wii Sports®, The Sims, and World of Warcraft (ESA, 2010). Some of the most popular games for children are music games such as Guitar Hero® and Rock Band®. These games provide opportunities for children to experience music, by making it. Thus, using Resnick's terms, they can be thought of as "pianos, not stereos."

A 2010 nationally representative survey of 2,002 third–12th grade students done by the Kaiser Family Foundation on children's media use found a significant increase in video gaming over the past 10 years, from an average of 26 minutes daily in 1999 to 49 minutes in 2004 and 73 minutes in 2009. According to the Kaiser Report (2010), this increase appears to be largely a function of the growing use of handheld devices for game playing. On any given day, 60% of young people play video games and spend an average of one hour and 13 minutes at it. Video game playing peaks among 11 to 14 year olds, especially for console playing. The Kaiser Report (2010) found that just as children begin to make the transition into adolescence, their media use explodes.

There remains a substantial difference between boys and girls in console video game playing, with boys spending an average of almost an hour a day playing and girls, just under 15 minutes. However, contrary to the public perception that media use displaces physical activity, young people who are the heaviest media users report spending similar amounts of time exercising or being physically active as other young people their age who are not heavy media users. So, while levels of physical activity do vary by age and gender, they don't vary by time spent using media (Kaiser Report, 2010).

Only a few years ago gaming was mostly viewed, in the best-case scenario, as a waste of time and most commonly as a risky activity that might lead to antisocial behavior, aggression, and violence, as well as reinforced gender stereotypes (Grüsser, Thalemann, & Griffiths, 2007). More recently, a growing body of research is starting to focus on "serious games" that might have a positive impact on young people (Squire & the Games-to-Teach Research Team, 2003). For example, there is increasing interest and expertise in developing serious computer games for promoting health (Kato, Cole, Bradlyn, & Pollock, 2008; Lieberman, 2001), education (Gee, 2007; Shaffer, 2007), and civic engagement (Bers, 2008c).

The 2008 Pew Internet and American Life Project report found that 44% of youth play games that teach them about a problem in society, while 52% play games that engage them in thinking about moral and ethical issues. The report also suggests that youth who have these kinds of civic gaming experiences are more likely to be civically engaged in the offline world and are also more likely to go online to get information about current events, try to persuade others how to vote in an election, become committed to civic participation, and raise money for charity.

Although public debate often frames video games as either good or bad, research shows that the context in which the video games are played and the content of the video games matter more than the amount of play time. Some video games might promote pro-social behavior and cognitive problem solving, while others might hinder them. Video games offer the opportunity to bring civic education back to life by engaging young people in simulations of political processes and immersing them in experiences in which making civic-based decisions are highly rewarded (Bers, 2010c). For example, researchers such as Squire and Barab (2004) have studied the positive learning impact of playing the historical simulation game Civilization.

Civilization was first developed in 1991 and has now been converted into a series with several sequels, such as Civilization II, Civilization III, Civilization IV, and Civilization Revolution, which present players with the goal to "build an empire to stand the test of time." The game begins in 4000 B.C., and the players attempt to expand and develop their empires through the ages by taking the role of rulers of a civilization and competing with other, already existing civilizations. For example, players need to explore far lands, judge when to engage in war or diplomacy, make decisions regarding when and where to build new cities, and decide which scientific and engineering advances can transform the cities to their maximum potential (Edwards, 2007). Later versions of this game allow for head-to-head play against other players.

Although video games might provide new opportunities for moral decision making and civic engagement, they might also obscure some of the intricacies of political decision making, which are hidden in the decisions made by game designers when conceiving game models that might be simple enough for simulations to work but do not take into consideration the complexities of political systems. Authoring kits that enable children to produce their own video games by modeling decision-making processes might yield better educational results in the long term. Once again, the child should be a producer, rather than a consumer. In this way, she has ample opportunity to develop competence as well as confidence.

Researchers such as Williams (2006a) suggest that the backdrop for the rise of social gaming is a decline in civic shared spaces for people to meet and converse face-to-face. Echoing Oldenburg's (1997) account of how third places—which are neither home nor work and cross-nationally might include social clubs, *tabernas*, piazzas, pubs, and public squares—are vital for community formation and maintenance, current research is showing that gaming, in particular virtual multiplayer games, might come to satisfy the human need for community and social interaction (Steinkuehler, 2006). Video game playing provides a space for social development and mastery of social relationships. Remember Erikson. From a developmental perspective, during the elementary school years, interactions with peers become more important than those with adults. This process continues its evolution into the teenage years.

Although video games are very popular, virtual worlds are becoming the most rapidly growing third places for children in elementary school. A 2008 report published by the Association of Virtual Worlds categorizes approximately 110 virtual worlds for kids, 115 for tweens, and 140 for teens. As of the second quarter of 2008, the largest virtual world for adults (over age 20) had 13 million registered users, while the largest for children had 90 million users (KZero Research, 2008). Virtual worlds such as Neopets (http://www.neopets.com/) are designed for children six to 12 years old. They can create their own Neopets by choosing their species, gender, and personality; set up their own shop; and feed them and look after them, as well as communicate with others, play games, and create their own Web pages. Children can also submit content for the weekly electronic newspaper called the *Neopian Times* and participate in a peer-based Neopets community. Children create artifacts and master new skills. On August 10, 2008, 237,138,604 Neopets had been created.

The eMarketer report found that of the 34.3 million U.S. child and teen Internet users, 24% in 2007, up to 34% in 2008, and 53% by 2011 visited virtual worlds once a month (Williamson, 2008). As an example of the increasing popularity of virtual worlds for children, the site Webkinz increased its visits by 1,141% in a year (Prescott, 2007), from less than one million to over six million (Tiwari, 2007). Club Penguin doubled in size, from 1.9 million to 4.7 million visitors (Shore, 2008). This popularity, however, is related to commercial endeavors. For example, Club Penguin was acquired by Disney, the popular Webkinz animals come with a code needed to enter the virtual world, and the Bratz fashion dolls are sold with a USB key necklace so the child can unlock the Be-Bratz.com virtual world (Beals & Bers, 2009).

These commercially focused virtual worlds and malls share many similarities. Their purpose is to sell products, to engage people in consuming different types of goods. We visit them, they are fun, they provide entertainment, and they satisfy our real or imaginary needs. They might become dangerous when we do not know how to handle ourselves in those spaces, when we cannot distinguish our needs from our desires. However, they bring to the forefront the importance of educating children. At the mall, parents might give children limited money and teach them what to buy and what to avoid. They might help them to select the appropriate stores; they might slowly teach them how to behave in a mall, how to avoid dangers, and how to take advantage of the best opportunities. Probably, parents do all this educational work without realizing it. Parents themselves are familiar with the mall. However, things are different in the virtual world. Parents might have never visited one, or they might not know what the best strategies for protecting their children are. Very few are familiar with Internet safety. Although there is a myriad of approaches developed by associations and nonprofit organizations, especially concerning the commercial nature of the Internet, parents might feel that their children are more vulnerable in a virtual world than in a commercial mall. The third part of the book will discuss this.

However, not all virtual worlds for children are commercially focused. For example, ZulaWorld.com, Quest Atlantis (Barab, Thomas, Dodge, Carteaux, & Tuzun, 2005; http://atlantis.crlt.indiana.edu/), River City (Dede, Ketelhut, Clarke, Nelson, & Bowman, 2005; Dede, Nelson, Ketelhut, Clarke, & Bowman, 2004; http://muve.gse.harvard.edu/river-cityproject/index.html), Second Life in Education (http://sleducation.wikispaces.com/), MOOSE Crossing (Bruckman, 1996; http://www.cc.gatech.edu/elc/moose-crossing/), Whyville (http://www.whyville.net/smmk/nice), 3DLearn (http://www.3dlearn.com/), Jumpstart (http://www.jumpstart.com/), and Zora (Bers, Chau, Satoh, & Beals, 2007; Bers, Gonzalez-Heydrich, & Demaso, 2001; http://ase.tufts.edu/devtech/tools.html), to name just a few, are designed with an explicit educational goal.

Are virtual worlds becoming the multimedia parks of the 21st century? If designed to support types of interactions similar to those that happen in the physical space and to promote the development of competencies, can they serve youth in a positive way? Subrahmanyam and Greenfield (2008) think so:

> For today's youth, media technologies are an important social variable and ... physical and virtual worlds are psychologically connected; consequently, the virtual world serves as a playing ground for developmental issues from the physical world, such as identity.
>
> (p. 124)

Are virtual worlds increasingly popular because they fulfill the need for spaces explicitly designed for the children in the older spectrum of the elementary years, the tween years, when issues of identity start to emerge? Sherry Turkle's pioneer work has proposed so. Back in 1995, she studied how the Internet could provide a "social laboratory" for exploring issues of identity. In the next chapter, I will discuss the role of technology in the high school years, when children are struggling to answer the question, "Who am I?"

Both parks and virtual worlds are carefully designed. Remember the landscape designer. She purposefully chooses the materials and arranges them to support a specific aesthetic or functional goal. The digital landscape for children, composed of virtual worlds, programming environments, and computer games, must promote positive development (Beals & Bers, 2010). In the elementary school years children are struggling with *industry* vs. *inferiority*, and they resolve this tension in a positive way by developing a sense of competence. New technologies must provide opportunities for children to become creators of digital projects and not just consumers, to learn new skills, and to share them with others (Barron, 2004).

Back in 1999, as part of my doctoral work at the MIT Media Lab under the direction of Seymour Papert, I developed the Zora virtual world. Inspired by the constructionist philosophy of learning, Zora provides easy-to-use tools for children to design and inhabit a virtual city. They can populate the virtual city by making their own virtual places and interactive creations, including 3-D objects, characters, message boards, and signs, as well as movies and sounds. Zora is a 3-D multiuser environment explicitly developed to provide a safe space for youth to explore issues of identity (Bers, 2001). The name *Zora* was inspired by one of the imaginary cities described by Italo Calvino (1972) as a city like a honeycomb in whose cells each person can place the things she wants to remember, so the world's most wise people are those who know Zora. My goal was to provide a space where children could become wise by knowing who they are—mastering their own selves.

Zora is a research-based virtual world. It has been used since 1999 in different pilot studies with several populations of young people, including those with end-stage renal disease undergoing dialysis treatment (Bers, Gonzalez-Heydrich, & DeMaso, 2001, 2003), multicultural groups (Bers, 2001; Bers & Chau, 2006), first-year students in college (Bers, 2008c; Bers & Chau, 2010), post-transplant pediatric patients (Bers et al., 2007; Bers, Lynch, & Chau, forthcoming), pediatric cancer patients in summer camps (Cantrell & Bers, 2010), and participants in national and international after-school computer-based learning centers (Beals & Bers, 2010). The vignettes and one of the case studies presented later share experiences from some of these projects.

Virtual environments are powerful platforms for developing educational programs. The potential of these immersive environments goes beyond the four walls of the classroom (Beals & Bers, 2009). As the physical and the virtual are becoming interconnected, it is important to understand how new technologies can be designed to best serve children's developmental needs. The fast-growing uses of virtual worlds for education are consistent with a recent paradigm change in the learning sciences—a change that is shifting the process of cognition from the head of one individual to a situated practice. As technology rapidly changes, new possibilities for crafting educational programs emerge. Thus, the question is: What will *not* change, when everything else changes? I believe that people's inclination to learn by doing rather than by being told won't change (Bers, 2009).

Multimedia parks in their many different forms—programming environments, video games, and virtual worlds—might provide children with opportunities to achieve mastery and competence as developmental milestones. At the same time, they can invite them to experiment with "what if" situations by making, creating, developing, discussing, and debating, as a way to explore their own identity. That is the major developmental milestone for the teenage years, which we will explore in the next chapter.

First the following vignettes will provide examples of how different kinds of technologies, such as the Zora virtual world, the Scratch programming language, and video games, engage elementary school–aged children in mastery and developing a sense of technological competence. The multimedia parks depicted in the next pages support children to become producers of digital projects, rather than just consumers.

Vignette 1
THE PERSONAL MEANING OF JUDAISM

By Marina Bers

Eliza, 12 years old, Cambridge, Mass.
Eliza is participating in a summer workshop using Zora to explore issues of identity in a multicultural setting. She lives in a wealthy part of town and is proud of her Jewish heritage. She wears necklaces with Jewish symbols around her neck and likes to read and write in Hebrew. She is driven, independent, and outgoing. She loves to talk about herself and has many friends. She has strong opinions about what is good and what is bad, and she is not shy to share them with others. Although she is not a technology geek, she quickly learns to navigate the Zora virtual city and to use its tools to create 3-D objects. But for her, the most interesting aspect of participating in the summer workshop is meeting other kids with different religious and cultural backgrounds. She attends a Jewish day school, so she welcomes the opportunity to participate in this summer multicultural workshop.

On the first day of the program, children are asked to create their own virtual homes and populate them with virtual objects to show the other children who they are. Zora's use of objects has been inspired by work that studied the meaning of the most cherished objects that people put in their homes (Csikszentmihalyi & Rochberg-Halton, 1981). These objects not only have a decorative function but also express people's value systems and personal identity.

In Zora, objects have properties that, besides defining their looks and functionality, also specify the meaning or personal and moral values that people assign to them. For example, a 12-year-old boy participating in the workshop created a greenhouse with pictures of bills from all over the world.

When he assigned the value "wealth" to a picture of a dollar and wrote, "I say that money is the symbol of material wealth. Its powers are vast but limited only to the material world," he was thinking about the meaning that money carries.

Eliza chose to build a virtual temple, instead of a personal home. She wasn't the only one to do so. Other kids also built a temple, such as Michael, who also built a TV room with his favorite shows. In the Jewish temple, Eliza created a 3-D Jewish prayer book with a blue cover, a sign with her name written in Hebrew letters, and an Israeli flag that flops around. She created yellow walls and a high ceiling. She also created two interactive characters using the Zora heroes function: Steven Spielberg and her dad, who is a rabbi. When clicked, each character tells a story about who he is and why he thinks Judaism is important.

In Eliza's Jewish temple, every object has a personal story linked to it as well as text aimed at teaching others about Judaism. For example, Eliza wrote the following description for the *kippah*: "Leather or cloth skullcap worn on the head to both show and feel closer connection to God through the body." When someone clicks on the *kippah*, it displays the following story written by Eliza:

> I live in the USA, and so I don't normally see Jews just walking down the street in a non-Jewish environment. Even if I did see one, I wouldn't know because Jews look the same as everyone else. That's why I love when I see someone in a kippah. They enable me to know if they are Jewish just by looking at them. I know it is not much, but whenever I see random people wearing kippot I feel closer to them. I know that being Jewish is just as important for them as it is to me.

Fourteen-year-old Axel connects to Zora. He creates an avatar, a virtual representation of himself, and a virtual home. A visit to Axel's home on Zora reveals much about the boy: his favorite colors, his most loved games, his family's history, and his friends. After working on his home, Axel navigates through the Baptist church, the French chateaux, and the sports arena. He first enters the Baptist church, and a priest welcomes him with a blessing. Alex finds this clever and decides to keep going around the virtual world. He enters Eliza's temple, and he clicks on a television that displays a snapshot from the movie *Schindler's List* that she found on the Web. He then clicks on the associated value, "documentation," and reads Eliza's definition:

> It is very important to remember history. That way, bad things won't happen again. Holocaust survivors are getting very old now, and if someone doesn't record their stories of what happened, we are doomed to forget and repeat the horrors.

While designing her Jewish temple Eliza explored Judaism, but even more important, she was able to reflect on what Judaism meant to her. She had the time and the space reserved for reflection and introspection. She wrote two or three stories for each object she created as well as many values and definitions. For example, Eliza chose the value "community" and linked it to a picture of her school yearbook. Here is her definition:

> At my school I don't just have teachers and classmates, everyone is friends. I hang out in the office with the staff or in the lounge with my peers. Whenever anyone has a problem, there is someone to whom we can go to for help. That is community.

During her experience in the workshop, Eliza started her journey interested in learning about other children's cultures and religions. However, as she worked on her own virtual space to teach others about Judaism, she realized that she was exploring what Judaism meant for her and her particular vision of it.

Vignette 2
DEVELOPING AS A COMPUTATIONAL CREATOR

by Karen Brennan

Anya, 14 years old, Eastern Europe.
Anya has loved the visual arts and drawing for as long as she can remember. She sketches on anything she can find and has dozens of sketchbooks, including sketches her mother saved from when she was very young. More recently, she has grown interested in how she can use her computer as a medium for drawing and sketching. She started using some basic paint editing tools but quickly graduated to professional tools like Photoshop and Illustrator.

Her uncle, who is a computer programmer, is supportive of Anya's artistic explorations with the computer and regularly gives her suggestions for new tools and techniques to try out. Anya's uncle discovered an article about the public debut of the Scratch Web site in May 2007. Scratch (http://scratch.mit.edu) is a programming environment designed for young people. It makes it easy to create interactive digital media—stories, games, simulations, animations, art—and then share those creations in an online community. Members can view each other's projects, engage in conversations, and download and remix each other's work. Anya's uncle saw Scratch as an opportunity to connect Anya's digital artistic interests with his programming interests.

After getting the recommendation from her uncle to try Scratch, Anya downloaded it and started tinkering with the sample Scratch projects. Starting with these as inspiration, she made different types of games—a collision-style game, a weather simulator, a greeting card—and shared her projects online. She was happy when other Scratchers in the community tried her projects and gave her feedback, and additionally, she made new friends on the site. She looked at other people's projects and experimented with remixing—downloading projects and extending them.

One thing she particularly likes to do with Scratch is to create animated sprites or characters. She thinks it is a nice way to bring her sketches to life. Other members were really impressed with her digital drawing abilities and started to make requests for other work. One girl asked Anya to create an animated sprite of a dragon breathing fire. A boy asked Anya to create an animated sprite of a cheetah running along a vast expanse of desert. More and more community members made requests for custom artwork—more than Anya could possibly handle. Inspired, she decided to create a Scratch tutorial project that explains step by step how to sketch different types of animals, objects, and characters.

Julie, a 10-year-old Scratcher from the United Kingdom, was impressed with Anya's Scratch projects and Anya's willingness to help others with their projects. Julie asked Anya if she would be interested in collaborating on a larger game project. Anya could create the artwork, another Scratcher could help with the game story line, another could help with some of the more complicated game programming, and Julie would manage and provide feedback on the collaboration. Anya was excited and agreed to join. She worked with Julie and a small team of Scratchers from around the world, ages 8 to 15, on a series of Scratch projects.

Anya's active participation and positive activities were noticed by the Scratch Team (MIT researchers who manage the Scratch Web site), and she was invited to serve as a moderator for the community. In this role, she is formally and publicly recognized as a Scratcher whom newer (and older) Scratchers can turn to with questions. She also gives suggestions to the Scratch Team about ways of improving the online Scratch community and the Scratch programming environment itself.

In her almost three years of engagement in the Scratch community, Anya has participated as a computational creator in a variety of ways: creating her own projects, supporting others' participation as computational creators, collaborating with others to make more elaborate projects, and acting as a moderator and mentor in the community of creators. Now 14 years old, she still uses Scratch to create interactive, dynamic computational media, but she also explores and experiments with other forms of digital expression.

Vignette 3
BEYOND SPORT

by Ashley Sandvi

Avery, 10 years old, Calhoun, Ga.

Avery, normally a reserved 10-year-old boy, becomes visibly exuberant when he talks about playing sports. A natural athlete, Avery recently completed his first season as quarterback of his county's 9- to 10-year-old tackle football team, the Longhorns. The team had had the same quarterback for three years, so earning the quarterback spot was a major victory for Avery. His first season was a winning one, and Avery loved having a leadership role on the team.

A love for sports is something Avery shares with his five siblings and stepsiblings. Before his parents' divorce, Avery was the oldest of three children. Three years ago, Avery's mother, Allison, married his stepfather, Thomas, who brought three children of his own to the relationship. So, in addition to Avery, there are five other children in this blended family: Austin, 17; Matthew, 15; Madison, 12; Bryson, 8; and Olyvia, 6.

The merging of the two families was relatively smooth, but each child had to find his or her own place in the new family. For Avery, it's very different being a middle child instead of the oldest. For Allison and Thomas, it's a challenge to make sure each child gets enough individual time and attention. Life is understandably hectic with six children under one roof, each of whom is active in sports and other activities. In addition to playing sports in real life, playing sports video games is a favorite pastime in Avery's home. His family has the Sony PlayStation 2 and the Nintendo Wii consoles, and the kids also have Nintendo DS handheld consoles, which come in handy while they are waiting for their siblings' sports practices to end.

Two of the games Avery plays most often are NCAA Football 09 on the PlayStation 2 and Madden NFL 10 on the Nintendo Wii. These video games offer somewhat realistic simulations of college and professional football games, respectively. Players can play by themselves against the computer, or they can play with their real-life friends. Both games are immensely popular. EA SPORTS has sold an astounding 85 million Madden games since 1988.

In addition to being entertaining, playing football video games allows players to learn about strategy. Playing the game increases overall knowledge of football, including defenses and coverage schemes, blocking patterns, and play action. Additionally, the video games allow players to establish an optimal level of challenge as they learn the game. Raising the difficulty level and practicing with the mini-game mode helps fine-tune players' strategy.

Avery feels that the time he spends playing football video games helped him earn the quarterback spot on his team. Though his strong throwing arm didn't hurt, Avery believes that the reason he earned the position is that he's the only player his coach trusts to remember all the plays. The ability to learn and practice plays through simulated video games makes them much easier for Avery to remember in real life. There are also more tactical benefits of playing football video games. In particular, Avery was excited to learn how to "juke" other players out—that's when he makes them think he's going one way but turns around and goes the other way to get a touchdown. Having the chance to practice bold plays in the simulated games makes him a more confident player in real life. He also says that the stretches he learned from the video games helped him increase his speed, which is important when he runs the ball.

Good quarterbacks must earn the trust of their team members, and playing football video games with other players on his team has been a fun bonding experience for Avery. The games allow players to play together on the same team or against each other as competitors. Playing football together using the video game helps Avery and his teammates develop a camaraderie that is different from that which develops during practice and real-life games. The close physical proximity while playing a video game allows the players to encourage each other and collaborate for an extended, uninterrupted period of time, as opposed to short bursts of time in a huddle on the field. Playing video games with his teammates helped Avery realize the importance of working together and encouraging each other. Now, Avery always makes an effort to encourage other players to get back up after being tackled and get back in the game. That's a life lesson that goes far beyond the football field.

CHAPTER 3

Wireless Hangouts vs. A Palace in Time During High School

This chapter focuses on the teen years of high school. By this age, young people are more interested in the act of getting together than the space in which they do so. Hanging out is a metaphor for spending time together, regardless of the location. The ubiquitous nature of wireless communication makes this possible. The metaphor of "wireless hangouts" captures adolescents' overwhelming need to be with others. However, this need is tied not to a physical space but to time. Teens want to spend times with other teens, not only because they enjoy it but also because being with others is a way to find out who they are themselves. This need to socialize responds to the major developmental milestone of the adolescent identified by Erikson, identity exploration. It doesn't happen in a social vacuum but, rather, in a constant exchange with others. The wireless hangout is a *no place* metaphor. However, wireless hangouts do not explicitly support purposeful identity exploration Therefore, in this chapter I juxtapose the metaphor of "wireless hangout" to the one of a "palace in time," another "no place" metaphor coined by the Jewish philosopher and theologian Abraham Joshua Heschel (1951) for describing the Sabbath. The Sabbath, the seventh day, is a palace in time for the Jewish people. It is a palace in time for identity. According to Heschel, it is the Sabbath that has kept the Jews as a people over so many generations, as opposed to the Jews having kept the Sabbath. Later in this section I will expand on this choice of metaphor, but for now it is enough to understand that, while wireless hangouts are important in adolescents' lives, some of those immersive experiences can become a palace in time to support their major developmental challenge: to quest for identity.

This generation of teenagers can meet online anytime and anywhere. However, today's teens struggle with issues of identity as much as past generations. Adolescence is a time to form a sense of individuality, to become aware of personal strengths and weaknesses. Teenagers start to realize that they can control their destinies but that they first need to define themselves and their goals. They are hungry for a sense of purpose in life, and they are likely to enroll in and support social causes.

According to Erikson (1963, 1982), adolescents experience *identity vs. role confusion*. As they transition from childhood to adulthood, they need to explore the question "Who am I?" while pondering the multiple roles they could play in the adult world. Adolescents know that the decisions they make now might have an impact on their future. They want to take their place in society, either by finding more or less conventional roles or by challenging established ways. At the same time, they need to find a sense of purpose, a stable and generalized intention to accomplish something that is at once personally meaningful and of consequence to the world (Damon, Menon, & Bronk, 2003).

Think of a 16 year old. He is studying hard because he wants to have good grades. Although he doesn't talk about it, he worries about college. After school, he plays in a band with other kids in the neighborhood. He spends hours practicing in basements. He has a favorite rock star and posters of him all over his room. Through his church, he volunteers tutoring inner-city children who are struggling in math. He is active in his school council and has made several proposals for changing school rules. During the summer, he works some weeks as a youth counselor at a summer camp and other weeks at a car wash. He is exploring different roles and ways of being. He gets into arguments with his parents, and he rebels against their worldviews. He thinks he knows it all, and he has the energy and conviction to change the world.

In the process of exploring identity, adolescents may experience role confusion, mixed ideas and feelings about different ways to be and to fit in society. A successful resolution of the tension *identity* vs. *role confusion* leads to the virtue of fidelity. Erikson defines it as the ability to sustain loyalties despite value systems that might be confusing and contradictory. Once a person has explored different ways of being and "what if" possibilities and has struggled with the confusion of belonging to multiple communities, she may reach a point when she feels that she has found herself. She has an emotional and deep awareness of who she is. She is able to adhere to her values, no matter how they might be challenged. In turn, this reinforces a continuing sense of identity.

Adolescence is characterized by the tension between differentiation and identification: the need to find boundaries between self and others, and the need for integration into a major whole consisting of family, culture, and society. Erikson talks about adolescence as a psychological moratorium, a "time out" when one can suspend decisions concerning long-term commitments and gain new experiences, encounter adventures, and experiment with multiple roles.

Sherry Turkle (1995), a psychoanalytically trained psychologist and sociologist, a professor at MIT, and a pioneer in studying people's personal relationship with technology, applied Erikson's concept of moratorium to the study of how adolescents use online environments as a social laboratory for experimenting with how the self is constructed and reconstructed in postmodern life. The pioneering work of Turkle has shown that technology serves to explore concepts of self as adolescents "cycle through" their own identities through playful experimentation.

Virtual worlds, among other online environments, may serve as spaces for moratorium. For example, the Habbo world (http://www.habbo.com/) is popular among adolescents. Habbo uses the metaphor of a hotel in which youth can meet others to play games and have fun. Users join this colorful, multidimensional virtual community and game environment by creating an online character or avatar called a Habbo (Beals, 2011). Users can design their avatars and their rooms and use furniture that can be purchased from a catalog. There is a code of conduct, called the "Habbo Way," that includes rules that users should adhere to, including, for example, not giving out passwords, not using hate speech, not telling people information about their location in real life, and not acting out violent acts. Habbo, along with other popular online environments, from virtual worlds to social networks, is an example of a wireless hangout for teenagers.

The metaphor of "wireless hangouts" captures adolescents' overwhelming need to explore who they are. This need is not tied to a physical space. The wireless hangout is a "no place" metaphor. Wireless hangouts are ubiquitous and popular among teenagers. However, they do not explicitly support purposeful identity exploration. In this chapter I juxtapose the metaphor of "wireless hangout" to the one of a "palace in time," coined by Heschel (1951) for describing the Sabbath. The Jewish tradition provides an interesting metaphor for thinking about what it means to explore identity, not casually in a wireless hangout but purposefully across time in a "no space."

Back in 1998, when first thinking about how to design virtual worlds to promote identity exploration, one image came to my mind: the Jewish Sabbath. According to Heschel, the seventh day belongs to the realm of time, as opposed to the realm of space. The Sabbath is a holy day that has been blessed by God in the story of Creation. I am not a strictly observant person, nor do I keep all the laws and rituals prescribed by Judaism with respect to the Sabbath. However, I find the idea of the

Sabbath fascinating. In a beautiful and simple manner, Heschel explored the many reasons that make the Sabbath a holy day. It is a time for introspection and reflection, a time for stopping everyday work and exploring who we are, how we are feeling, and how we may participate in our community (Bers, 2008d).

This notion has some similarities with Erikson's moratorium. Researchers following in Turkle's pioneering steps found that adolescents experience this search for identity in different wireless hangouts and through many ways (Calvert, 2002; Subrahmanyam, Greenfield, Kraut, & Gross, 2001). According to a 2010 Pew Internet and American Life Project report, 93% of teens ages 12 to 17 go online. Once there, they do different things. Nearly three-quarters (73%) of online teens visit social network sites. The older online teens, ages 14–17 (82%), use online social networks more than younger teens ages 12 and 13; 8% of online teens visit virtual worlds like Gaia, Second Life, or Habbo Hotel; 62% of online teens get news about current events and politics online; 48% bought books, clothing, or music online; 31% of online teens get health, dieting, or physical fitness information from the Internet; and 17% gather information online about topics that are hard to discuss with others, such as drug use and sexual health.

The report also notes that Internet connectivity is increasingly moving off the desktop into the mobile and wireless environment. Access to the Internet is changing. Although 93% of teens use a computer to go online, they also use cell phones, game consoles, and portable gaming devices to access the Internet. Some 75% of American teens ages 12–17 have a cell phone, and more than a quarter (27%) use them to go online. Similarly, 24% of teens with a game console (like a PlayStation 3, Xbox, or Wii) use it to go online (Lenhart et al., 2008). Internet access is becoming ubiquitous for young people. But wireless hangouts go beyond. The report shows that text messaging has become the primary way that teens reach their friends anywhere, anytime.

Despite technology being ubiquitous and the digital landscape easy to access, not all online environments are conducive to support purposeful explorations of identity. Not all wireless hangouts can become a palace in time. In my own work, I have explicitly designed several environments to support this developmental process, Zora being one of them (Bers, 2001). When I was designing them, the images associated with the Sabbath came to mind.

The seventh day served me as a powerful object to think with (Papert, 1980). It illuminated the kind of experience that I hoped young people would have while engaging with the technology. I imagined them entering into a palace in time where they would find tools for self-reflection and community building. I hoped teens would collaborate with others in ongoing community projects and in the process explore their sense of self, purpose, and belonging. I provided them with tools that went beyond the traditional prayers, words, and conversations that I found at the synagogue. I wanted the results of quiet introspection and self-reflection to become tangible and manipulable. Thus in Zora children can create virtual temples with interactive objects and characters that express values and stories. And they can program virtual objects to react to user inputs. Zora, as an example of a palace in time, affords similar experiences to the ones I personally had when observing the Sabbath: self-reflection, creation, creativity, communication, and participation in a community.

While other virtual hangouts, such as Teen Second Life and social networking sites such as Facebook, might also support this developmental need, Zora was developed as a research platform with a theoretical and pedagogical framework, Positive Technological Development, that looks at the positive role that technology can play in young people's lives. The second part of the book will present the components of the PTD framework. PTD guides the design of digital landscapes that can serve similar developmental functions as playgrounds in early childhood, parks in the elementary school years, and a palace in time during adolescence.

First, the following vignettes present different examples of how the wireless hangout may become a palace in time to explore issues of identity and connect with others. The examples show how high school teenagers develop and make their mark in the online world through posting on YouTube to showcase their unique skills, building connections with people in games like World of Warcraft (virtually and physically), and making connections around the world by simply sharing their passion.

Vignette 1
15 MINUTES OF FAME

By Clement Chau

Ty Moss, 18 years old, North Carolina.
UrbanDictionary.com describes Ty Moss as "the awesome guy on *YouTube* who has cool tech videos and awesome daily vlogs" (http://www.urbandictionary.com/define.php?term=Ty%20Moss). Ty is an 18-year-old YouTube personality who is known for his short video clips about iPhone and other Apple Inc. products and gadgets on the YouTube channel tysiphonehelp. Starting when he was 16, Ty has produced over 500 video clips distributed across five

different YouTube channels. Many of these video clips feature his comments and reviews about the newest gadget on the market, while others are about his life and hobbies. With over 120,000 subscribers and video clips reaching as many as 30 million view counts each, Ty Moss is viewed in the new media advertising industry as the epitome of viral marketing. Many new media technology companies send samples for Ty to review, and others aggressively seek a quick mention by him in a video. In return, Ty receives perks from various companies and financial compensation for embedding advertisements in his video clips. For Ty, YouTube is not only a source of social networking but also a source of income. For his audience, Ty is a perfect example of how young people are finding ways to craft a niche in the new media landscape to express their interests and ideas while making a significant impact on the market, the arts, and the economy.

YouTube provides a platform for anyone with a consumer-level digital video camera an opportunity to create video clips to share with the world. As a user-generated content platform, YouTube provides mechanisms for users to share content; the YouTube staff does not create any original video content and does little to monitor, manage, or advertise the content created by its users. After a simple registration process, anyone over the age of 13 can create an account and a channel page to distribute video clips and monitor audience reaction via a rating and feedback comment system. Audience members can add particular video clips to their Favorites play lists and subscribe to a favorite user's channel to receive updates when a new video clip is posted. In these ways, YouTube creates a community around sharing video clips.

Ty Moss is one of many teens who have found YouTube as a new media playground. Ty loves playing with the newest technology and electronic gadgets, and he is someone we might call a tinkerer and a little bit of a hacker. At the age of 16, Ty received an iPhone, a popular smart cellular phone produced by Apple. Promptly after receiving the iPhone, Ty learned of a way to unlock or hack the system of the phone so that he could use unauthorized features and applications on his new gadget. At that time, Ty was also engrossed with the YouTube culture, where amateurs post video clips of all kinds of topics. He made his debut video quickly after he learned of the hack feature and posted the video *The Easiest Way to Jailbreak ANY Firmware iPhone!* on his newly created channel on February 15, 2008. This video received 500 viewers within a single day; within two weeks it was indexed and searchable by the Google search engine; and by May 14, 2009, his debut video made it to the list of Featured Videos on the YouTube front page. To date, Ty's debut video has over 37,000 views, and it launched his career as a YouTube personality known for his videos on topics related to technology and new media.

Ty has learned over time that being a YouTube personality can be a career; but it is not an easy one. Ty has learned to manage business (creating an online store to sell merchandise related to his celebrity), build a relationship with his audience (via Twitter, Facebook, and live video chats), control advertising and revenue streams (via the YouTube Partner program, whereby he profits from advertisements embedded in his videos), and liaise with the new technology and gadget industry partners so that he can be first to review their products on YouTube. When asked, Ty would quickly say that YouTube is his main occupation, and one in which he works hard to maintain his significance within the community and to ensure that he remains a top search result when anyone looks for tips and trends related to Apple products. To this end, he has created numerous Web sites, attended industry events, and kept up to date with the newest innovations and trends in the market. In other words, Ty works to maintain relevance and dominance over a niche that he created within the YouTube community to make certain that his *15 minutes of fame* lasts longer than 15 minutes.

Today, Ty has branched out to review and "blog" about other gadgets and applications such as game console systems, software applications, and new media trends. He created other channels including tyistech and tyonthefly to accommodate video content not related to the iPhone or Apple. In addition, Ty connects with his audience through his personal channel, 0TyMoss0, where he produces video blogs, or vlogs, about his day-to-day life. His fans and subscribers watch Ty report about his day—whether it is a video clip about his new girlfriend; a trip to the hair salon; his annoying sister; or Ty getting ill, then well, then ill again. Through these video clips, the audience learns about not only Ty's perspectives on the newest gadgets but also who Ty is as a teenager. The audience provides Ty support and motivation to produce new video clips, and in return, Ty responds to technical questions raised by the audience. This dynamic relationship helps sustain Ty's interests in the community and gives him inspiration and ideas to create more video clips that his audience would enjoy watching. Beyond contributing to the YouTube community and helping his audience, Ty also leverages his celebrity to promote charity work, such as his participation in Project for Awesome, in which he encouraged his audience to donate to the Lumos charity (then called the Children's High Level Group). Nonetheless, aside from the range of personal video clips Ty has made over the years about his life, his passion and his niche remain Apple Inc. products.

Vignette 2
A WORLD OF ONE'S OWN

by Lauren Lanster

Jen, 16 years old, Mattapoissett, Mass.
Jen is a shy 16-year-old high school student from Mattapoissett, Massachusetts, who lives somewhat far from her friends and from his boyfriend of just under

a year. She is a high school junior and is having difficulties coping with how far her home is from her high school and friends, as she lives about an hour away by car and does not have her driver's license. She recently moved into her house in Mattapoissett and does not know many people there.

Her father is the CEO of a company and constantly works until late at night and travels. Her mother lives with her younger brother, a golf prodigy, in Florida, where she can supervise his golf trips. Though her parents are not divorced or separated, the whole family is rarely together except for a weekend every six weeks or so. Jen's boyfriend, whom she met at a summer program, lives in Miami, Florida, and she sees him once a month at best. Thus, Jen finds herself home alone a lot of the time.

To cut the loneliness and pass the time after school until her father comes home, Jen has started playing World of Warcraft (WoW), a massively multi-player online role-playing game (MMORPG) launched in November 2004 by Blizzard Entertainment. With more than 12 million subscribers as of October 2010, WoW is currently the world's most-subscribed MMORPG (http://us.blizzard.com/en-us/company/press/pressreleases.html?101007). As with other MMORPGs, players create and control a character avatar within a game world, explore the landscape, fight various monsters, complete quests or missions that can bring rewards, interact with nonplayer characters or other players, and form and join guilds. While a character can be played on its own, players can also group with others to tackle more challenging quests. As characters become more developed, they can gain various talents and skills and learn different professions.

Initially, Jen only devoted one or two hours a week to the game, but she soon found herself having more and more fun playing. She especially liked to go on "kills" with other players, in hopes of killing bosses. Players acquire possessions, called loot, during these "kills," and the more possessions one owns, the better. Jen found herself accumulating more and more possessions and finding her skill level rising sharply.

Jen became such a good player that she quickly rose in the ranks and started being scouted out by other players to join their guilds. She stopped dreading the long hours home alone without her family and started embracing her virtual family. Like a real-life family, she and other players would look out for each other during "raids" and schedule times to meet online during the day. She introduced the game to some of her friends at school, so they could play together while being far apart from each other. By signing into her WoW account, the one-hour geographical distance between Jen and her friends became obsolete. She found herself becoming closer with her school friends, especially the males.

Jen began mediating a forum about WoW where people posted hints, asked for help, gave advice, and shared other facts about "killing bosses" and acquiring goods in WoW. People sought her advice. At 16, Jen was helping players all around the world, some of whom were over twice her age. Jen eventually took a trip to California to BlizzCon, a large annual convention for games released by Blizzard. She wanted to meet her virtual family that so often substituted for her real family. The connection became even stronger, and Jen made long-lasting friendships with the people she spent several hours a day online with.

After about a year, Jen's school work began to suffer. Jen realized this and sold her account. However, she still maintains an administrative status on the forums and continues to give advice to those struggling to succeed in WoW. She keeps the virtual friendships she made but also has stronger connections with her school friends. WoW facilitated a way for Jen to hang out with her friends despite the difficulty of the geographical distance between her home and school. Without such a platform, Jen might not have learned the value of collaborating with others in the pursuit of the same goal and working in a team environment. Though her school work did start to suffer, she learned how to deal with the responsibility of filling a role in a group and communicating with others. For a shy 16 year old, this was an education unlike any other.

Vignette 3
A GLOBAL CONNECTION

By Alyssa Ettinger

Ricky, 17 years old, London.
Ricky has excelled at football (soccer) since his first five-a-side game at age three. His natural talent and strong kick earned him the nickname "Golden Foot" by his first coach. Having lived in London all his life, Ricky worked his way up to play on the Watford youth team, one of several club teams in the football-mad city looking to gather talented young players. As a junior in high school, Ricky is not quite good enough to play professionally, so he is now exploring universities that would allow him to continue playing at a slightly less rigorous caliber. He is interested in the London School of Economics, which could satiate his growing fascination with business and entrepreneurship, as well as allow him to join the football team.

A dedicated and inquisitive student, Ricky has developed a great appreciation for the strategy and philosophy behind the game to add to an impressive repertoire of technique and footwork. He enjoys watching international games year-round, intently studying the subtle skills and player formations modeled by the professionals. Years of watching games, researching players, and learning from his own football experiences have resulted in a vast, multidimensional network of insights into the sport. Last summer, Ricky was inspired to express and share this passion for football by creating a blog on a social networking site, Tumblr. The micro-blogging site offers an easy-to-use interface with customizable colors, themes, and layouts. Users can create and publish text, photo, audio, and video content, which is viewed and often "reblogged" by other users, instantly passing on content while crediting the author.

Ricky spent weeks choosing the perfect background pictures, font colors, and layout for his blog and even created a logo with the tagline "Colorful insight on the world's greatest game." Eventually, he began posting his own football news stories, live blog updates on current games, editorials, and other witty perspectives on the sport, complete with YouTube video links to related interviews and game clips when appropriate. As fellow Tumblr users read, commented on, and reblogged Ricky's posts, Ricky rapidly garnered a relatively large global audience. About one year after his blog's creation, he was featured as "Tumblr's Favorite Sports Site" in the directory and has since received overwhelmingly positive feedback from his readers. Ricky takes great pride in looking up his site traffic statistics using Google Analytics, proof that his content is being read by people in over 100 countries.

As his site has grown, Ricky has been able to take advantage of his widespread audience to raise awareness for various international charities, categorized under his "Good Causes" tab. He provides a link to the charities' Web sites and a short editorial for each one, encouraging donations from readers. Ricky is currently exploring ways to make his site more interactive by negotiating deals with football merchandizing Web sites and creating contests for readers to enter with a "free giveaway" prize. He has even begun to receive advertising offers from football and other sports-based companies, opening the doors for a promising entrepreneurship opportunity before even entering university. Ricky now corresponds daily with other young football-loving readers from around the world who are fans of his blog. Most recently, some readers have contacted Ricky with the hopes of contributing to his site as student-writers. To Ricky's surprise, they are willing to write for free. Indeed, the blog's success provides for valuable publicity for such young writers, not to mention a powerful asset on their college résumés.

Summary

This summary provides an overview of the key ideas in the first part of the book. The introduction presented the need for the PTD framework, from both a personal perspective and an academic one. It also provided a description of this theoretical model and the two main intellectual traditions from which it was conceived, Constructionism and positive youth development. The first part of the book introduced the notion of technology as a developmental space. By using Erikson's psychosocial framework, which focuses on the struggles and milestones at different developmental stages, I used different metaphors to think about the role of technology as supporting the fundamental tasks for positive development at different age ranges. Table PI:1 summarizes these chapters.

Table PI.1: Spatial Metaphors in the Digital Landscape

	Early Childhood (2–5 Years Old)	Elementary School (6–12 Years Old)	High School (13–17 Years Old)
Developmental tension	Autonomy vs. shame and doubt	Industry vs. inferiority	Identity vs. role confusion
Developmental milestone or virtue	Will power Purpose	Mastery of new skills Competence	Fidelity Loyalty
Metaphors	Playgrounds vs. playpens Playgrounds support autonomous explorations, creativity, open-ended play, risk taking. Child can choose and is in control. Playpens are safe and support limited exploration and creativity. Adult chooses and is in control.	Parks vs. malls Parks afford mastery of multiple skills. Child can choose. The child is in the role of creator. Malls are limited in the types of competencies they can support. Commercialism. The child is in the role of consumer.	Wireless hangouts vs. palace in time Wireless hangouts allow connection with peers anywhere, anytime. May be used to explore identity. Palace in time is explicitly designed to support identity formation and exploration.

PART II

A Framework for Designing Digital Landscapes for Personal Development

OVERVIEW

The first part of the book focuses on how our digital landscape can best serve developmental needs at different ages. This second part explores how to purposefully design digital experiences to support positive youth development. What are the design elements that need to be taken into consideration for empowering personal and community growth? What kinds of behaviors should our technological landscape support? How do we integrate what we know is best, from the point of view of children's development, with the design affordances of the technologies? While the first part of the book took a descriptive approach, this one takes an interventionist one. The focus is on design. Most specifically, it is on the design of technologically rich experiences to promote positive youth development. There is intentionality and value judgment regarding the best digital spaces for our children. We need to remember that, unlike the natural landscape, our digital landscape is a designed space.

Design is about making choices informed by constraints. It is about creative approaches to solve problems; it is about following our intuition and recognizing patterns. It requires empathy and emotional connection with those who will become users of the products, experiences, and processes we are designing. Design is a human-centered rather than a technology-centered activity. Designing developmentally appropriate digital landscapes involves matching developmental needs, available technologies, and constraints of the sociocultural context. As you read this, you might start to think: "I am not a designer," "I don't have technological skills," "I don't know how to make things."

Don't worry. There is a difference between *being* a designer and *thinking* like a designer (Brown, 2009). Design thinking is about design with a "small d." It moves away from the concept of design associated with grandiose objects displayed at modern art museums, efficient software that solves unthinkable problems, and everyday engineering marvels. Design thinking is about a creative, human-centered exploration that is willing to embrace competing constraints. Digital landscapes for young people have developmental constraints. According to Tim Brown, CEO and president of IDEO, design thinking is an approach to creative problem solving informed by three mutually reinforcing elements: insight, observation, and empathy.

As designers of technological landscapes that support positive youth development, we need insight to identify the developmental tasks that children face while growing up. In the previous chapters I referred to them as the developmental tensions identified by Erik Erikson, with their positive resolution in the form of virtues or desired milestones. For example, a 10 year old who is encountering issues of industry vs. inferiority might benefit from digital experiences that are different from those needed by a teenager who is going through identity vs. role confusion. Insight comes from academic knowledge but also from going out into the world and observing people's behaviors. By spending time with young people and observing how they use technology we can assess what developmental needs are met and which ones are not. What kind of developmental processes is the technology facilitating, replacing, augmenting, and hiding? Remember, we are thinking about design as a human activity, centered on the individual, not on the technology.

Insight and observation can tell us a lot about the developmental needs of our children and the technological constraints of the digital landscape. However, we are not only anthropologists studying children; we want the best for them. Here is where the third element of design thinking comes into place: empathy. Our ability to stand in children's shoes, to connect with them, will allow us to translate our observations and insights into decisions that will improve their experiences in the digital landscape. We know that it is a complex, confusing, and contradictory world. We need children's guidance to show us the issues they are struggling with and to orient us to possible solutions. We need them to become design thinkers as well. Tim Brown, when talking to business leaders who want to become design thinkers, uses this language:

> We need to invent a new form of collaboration that blurs the boundaries between creators and consumers. It is not about "us versus them" or even "us on behalf of them." For the design thinker, it has to be "us with them."
>
> (2009, p. 58)

Allison Druin, who works on the design of novel human–computer interfaces, refers to this as participatory design experiences. In her methods, she (2002) always includes children as co-designers.

You are probably wondering how you will address some of children's needs if you cannot change the technology itself or you cannot build new software or hardware. Remember, it is not about the object itself but, rather, about the uses we give to that object, about the range of experiences it supports. Fortunately for us, this digital landscape is so vast and rich that it has many things to offer. We don't always need to build new technologies ourselves to make the best design choices to support positive youth development.

My own academic path started as a designer of new technologies at the MIT Media Lab. However, over the years I learned that designing the context of usage of those technologies, the scenarios, is as important as the design of the tools. For example, a well-planned curriculum in a well-managed classroom can complement the design affordances of most technologies. When working with robotics and young children, there is nothing in the design of the robots themselves that prompts children to collaborate with each other. However, a curriculum that engages them in cooperative activities, a classroom setup that favors conversations around small tables, and a teacher who invites children to help each other will be on target to meet young children's developmental need of learning to work with others. As long as we know the kinds of behaviors that we want our technological landscape to support and promote, we can become landscape designers of our digital world. We can choose, we can adapt, we can restrict, we can complement. There is a vast offering of technologies to choose from. But we need a framework to guide our choices. Positive Technological Development is such a framework.

This second part of the book is organized in six chapters that correspond to each of the six C's of the PTD theoretical framework. The first three chapters address the C's that are most relevant to supporting behaviors that will enrich the intrapersonal domain (content creation, creativity, and choices of conduct, which in turn promote personal assets such as competence, confidence, and character). The last three chapters address the interpersonal domain. They look at social and civic aspects (communication, collaboration, and community building and the corresponding caring, connection, and contribution). Each chapter presents the core concept and makes connections to academic disciplines that have addressed it in more depth. It is not the goal of this book to dive into each of these C's with scholarly depth—multiple books can be written about each one of them—but, rather, to provide an overview while highlighting how all of the C's are interconnected. The key is the overall framework, the relationships between the C's, the need for all of them "to help children learn new things to become better people and make a better world." Remember? That was the original goal that led me to undertake this academic journey. Each chapter in part II of the book, alongside with the academic discussion, provides examples from my own work of over a decade and a half designing technologically rich environments to promote positive youth development. Each chapter is followed by several vignettes with examples from our technological landscape across the developmental span. At the end of the second part, a summary reviews the main ideas.

CHAPTER 4

Creating Digital Content to Promote Competence

The first C of the PTD framework, content creation, is the most powerful of all: our technological landscape must provide opportunities for children to create their own projects. This involves a fundamental switch in the role of the child with regards to digital content: children as producers, as opposed to consumers (Bers, 2010d). As children grow, their ability to create content might also grow with the use of more sophisticated technologies.

For example, a four year old with the developmental need of exploring issues of autonomy to develop a sense of will power might benefit from working with developmentally appropriate software that provides opportunities to show the results of his efforts in a simple way. The four year old needs a technological playground where he can take the initiative and make a project. The nature of the project, the final outcome, is not as important as the process of creating it. This journey builds self-esteem, as children can proudly say, "I did it!" A nine year old who is navigating the developmental tension of industry vs. inferiority will build on this developmental trajectory, but the focus will be on mastery and learning of new skills (i.e., competence in the technological domain) not only on playful explorations. A teenager who is exploring issues of identity might be inclined to create content by participating in social media and playing online simulation games to explore aspects of herself. All of these experiences allow children and youth to participate in the digital landscape as content creators.

That is the basic tenet of Constructionism. The PTD framework builds on this and suggests that the possibilities of creating with new technologies promote not only learning but also positive development. A child who can create projects will develop a sense of competence, a sense of mastery.

And like a chain reaction, the more competence a child has, the more she will be able to do, which sharpens her skills and leads her to become even more competent (Bers, 2010d).

Research focused on children as digital content producers spans two different areas. The first is advocated by Papert's constructionist tradition, which follows on Piaget's theories. As we have seen in previous chapters it focuses on computer programming as a mechanism to produce content. Over the years, from Logo to Scratch, different programming environments have been developed for children. The second area is advocated by researchers who focus on new media literacies as a mechanism for producing content. In this view, children should develop skills and competency in the participatory practices of the online world (Jenkins, Purushotma, Clinton, Weigel, & Robison, 2006). In the following paragraphs, we will examine both approaches to content creation, the one proposed by the constructionist tradition and the one suggested by the new media literacies group. We will start with Constructionism, as it is my intellectual home.

Constructionism suggests that one of the best ways to engage children in digital content creation is through teaching them computer programming. Although some might think of computer programming as textual code, complicated algorithms, and geeks working all night long, the interfaces for computer programming have drastically changed. We can program computers by telling stories, dragging and dropping icons, and sequencing different graphics. Much of the work done in the constructionist tradition has focused on developing user-friendly programming environments that even young children can learn how to use. Programming uses the full potential of the computer, as opposed to limiting it to a powerful typewriter, fast calculator, or instant mail service. Programming adds interactivity to the content that we create, but most important, it engages us in developing technological fluency, the ability to express ourselves through technology.

The concept of technological fluency invites us to see beyond a traditional approach that positions the computer as an "instrumental machine." Computers, particularly when one is capable of programming them, can become epistemological machines that help us "think about thinking" in new ways. Jeannette Wing, a computer science professor at Carnegie Mellon University, coined the term *computational thinking* to refer to this kind of competence. She describes computational thinking as a fundamental skill for everyone, not just for computer scientists:

> To reading, writing, and arithmetic, we should add computational thinking to every child's analytical ability. Just as the printing press facilitated the spread of the three

R's, what is appropriately incestuous about this vision is that computing and computers facilitate the spread of computational thinking. Computational thinking involves solving problems, designing systems, and understanding human behavior, by drawing on the concepts fundamental to computer science. (2006)

Computational thinking refers to a range of mental tools, found in the breadth of the field of computer science, that involve analytical thinking. Thus, computational thinking shares similarities with mathematical thinking (e.g., problem solving), engineering thinking (designing and evaluating processes), and scientific thinking (systematic analysis). The foundation is abstraction—abstracting concepts from cases and evaluating and selecting the "right" abstraction. It relies on selection of inputs (manipulation of variables and computational instructions), observation of outputs (outcome data), and decomposition of what happens in between. Computational thinking involves the ability to abstract from specific programming languages the computational behaviors that can be implemented through many different languages. For example, a child who learns to program in Logo, and masters not only the specific syntax of the Logo program but the computational ways of thinking required to create a project (for example, she understands when to use variables), is likely to learn a new programming language without much difficulty. She will need to master the new syntax, but she will have already learned how to think in computational ways. She will have mastered the fundamental concepts of computer science; she will be able to identify potential "bugs" and places for errors, to decide what details among the input-computation-output algorithm to highlight and retain and what details to discard.

When children program interactive projects, they engage in a series of interrelated multiple steps that might or might not be linear. They identify a final goal, they formulate an action plan, they make an initial attempt to meet their goals, they test and evaluate, they revise their ideas by assessing what went wrong and what they could do better, and they formulate new attempts to compensate for failure (Bers, 2010b; Bers & Horn, 2010). This iterative experience engages them in what engineers call the engineering design process, computer scientists call the software development cycle, and researchers in the field of human development call intentional self-regulation.

Regardless of the disciplinary vocabulary, a child engaged in this design process is building internal capacities associated with competence in the technological domain. But she might also use this iterative process when writing a poem, solving a mathematical equation, or developing a scientific experiment. This set of complex and abstract metacognitive processes is sometimes referred to in the literature as executive functions that enable self-regulated learners to set goals, strategize, and self-monitor in order to process the information around them (Blair, 2002). These are all factors in a child's ability to succeed in school and within interpersonal relationships with teachers and peers (Biermann & Pattberg, 2008).

Competence is not an innate asset; it can be built and reinforced when provided with opportunities. Researchers and practitioners inspired by the constructionist tradition provide those opportunities by developing different kinds of programming languages for children. Constructionists believe that to benefit from the computer as a "tool to think with" children need to learn how to program. For example, Andy diSessa, a professor of cognition and development at the University of California, Berkeley, says that cutting off programming is like cutting off half the power of the computer medium—like reading without writing (Soloway, 1993). However, what kinds of programming environments are we designing? Upon which metaphors are they built? Does our digital landscape offer a vast array of opportunities? These are fair questions; until very recently most of the work in this area tended to only attract those who were comfortable with mathematical ways of thinking.

The Logo programming language developed by Seymour Papert and colleagues used the metaphor of a turtle that follows directions to move on the computer screen. How far and in which direction the turtle moves are described by numbers. Later on, the inclusion of graphics and multimedia expanded Logo's capabilities (see Figure 4.1). However, Logo was explicitly designed to immerse children in math land.

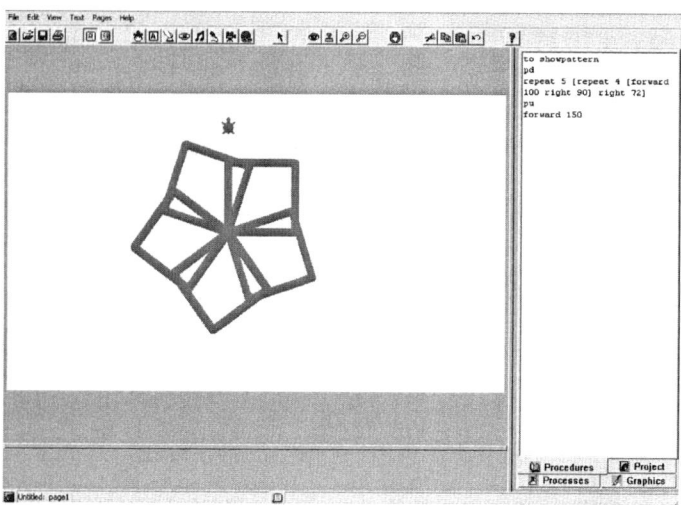

Figure 4.1. The Logo programming language.

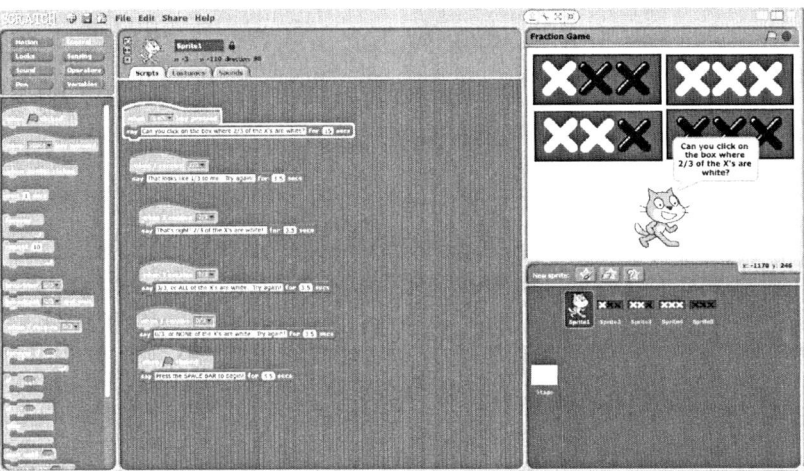

Figure 4.2. The Scratch programming language.

More recently, the Scratch programming language, developed by Mitchel Resnick and colleagues at the MIT Media Lab, uses the metaphor of characters, called "sprites," on a performing stage. Using a graphical language, and not just child-friendly syntax as Logo did, children put together blocks that fit like a puzzle to give commands to the sprites (see Figure 4.2). A useful metaphor to understand Scratch is to think about the child as a stage director who gives commands to different characters by putting together a puzzle to tell a story.

The puzzle metaphor is powerful for visual programming languages that engage children. At Tufts University, Mike Horn, a former student of mine and now teacher at Northwestern University, developed as part of his doctoral dissertation the Tern programming language (Horn & Jacob, 2007). Tern extends the puzzle concept to the physical world. Rather than using a keyboard or mouse to write programs on a computer screen, children use a collection of interlocking wooden blocks to build physical computer programs to control a robot's behavior. Each block represents an action, a flow-of-control construct, a parameter, or a sensor value. Tern uses computer vision to convert the physical programs into digital code (Horn, Bers, & Jacob, 2009).

Later on, based on Horn's work on Tern, and with funding from the National Science Foundation, other students in my DevTech research group, Jordan Crouser and David Kiger, extended Tern to become the CHERP hybrid system specifically aimed at early childhood. CHERP has both a tangible or physical component (interlocking wooden blocks that represent elements of a simple programming language for controlling robots) and a graphical element (the same icons appear as part of an on-screen tool palette of "virtual blocks"). In CHERP, both virtual blocks and wooden blocks represent the same robotic instructions (see Figure 4.3). The physical characteristics of the wooden blocks are designed to make syntax errors virtually impossible: if two icons do not fit syntactically, the blocks will not fit physically. Similarly, the virtual blocks will only "snap together" to form a program in a syntactically appropriate sequence. The metaphor of selecting blocks and connecting them together to form a program remains constant in both interfaces. Children can freely switch between interfaces to program their robots. This hybrid approach provides young children with the opportunity to create content using multiple representations (Horn et al., 2011).

Many programming environments for children have been created over the years by researchers in different academic institutions and are at different stages of development. Each one uses a different metaphor. For example, AgentSheets, first developed by Alex Repenning in 1999 at the University of Colorado, is designed for middle and high school students to create Web-based simulation games. Similar to a spreadsheet, an "agentsheet" is a computational grid. However, unlike spreadsheets, this grid does not just contain numbers and strings but, rather, so-called agents represented by pictures that can be animated,

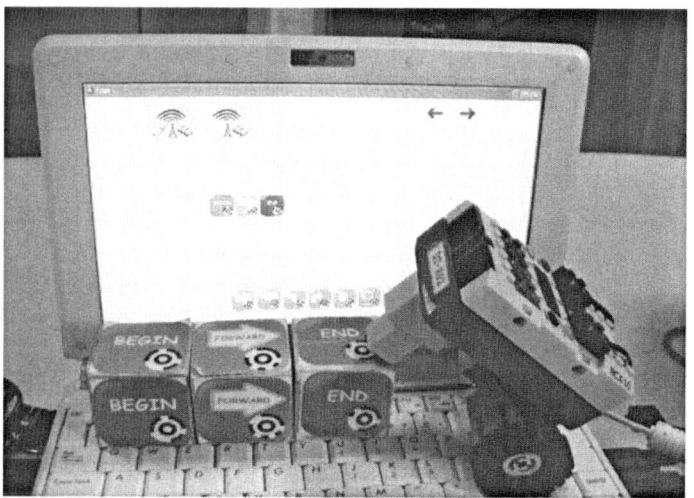

Figure 4.3. The CHERP hybrid programming language.

make sounds, react to mouse/keyboard interactions, read Web pages, speak, and even recognize speech commands (Repenning, Webb, & Ioannidou, 2010).

Alice, developed at Carnegie Mellon University, is a 3-D programming environment for middle and high school students to learn about object-oriented programming. It uses 3-D graphics and a drag-and-drop interface to facilitate the creation of animated movies and simple video games. In Alice, 3-D objects (e.g., people, animals, and vehicles) populate a virtual world, and students create a program to animate the objects. By manipulating the objects in their virtual world, students gain experience with all the programming constructs typically taught in an introductory programming course.

In my early work at the MIT Media Lab, I developed the Storytelling Agent Generation Environment (SAGE), an authoring environment for children to create their own wise storytellers to interact with by telling and listening to stories (Bers, 2003a; Bers & Cassell, 1998). The environment allows children to model the conversational flow between user and storyteller by selecting and arranging graphical objects such as turn-taking states, communicative actions, and parts of conversation (see Figure 4.4). Children create conversational flows in the same way that they engage in pretend role-play games, by planning who is going to say what and when. They also create a database of inspirational stories that the storyteller could tell in response to a user's problems.

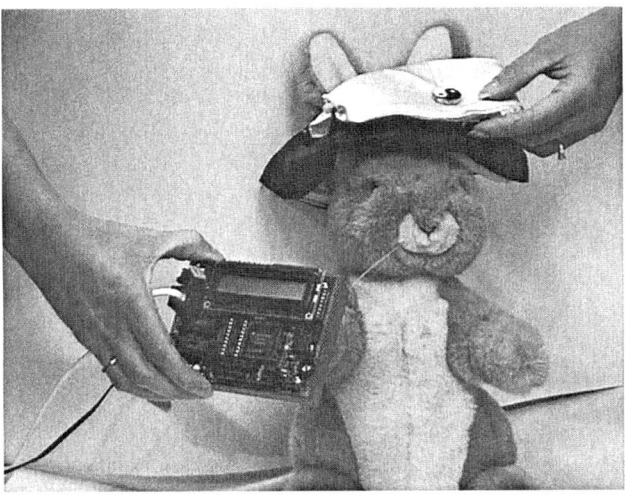

Figure 4.4. The SAGE interface composed of a robotic stuffed toy.

In my research with SAGE, I found that children were able to design and model abstract structures needed and used in both programming and storytelling. They created, manipulated, and put together narrative building blocks such as speaker turns, scripts, and communicational actions. In the process they used programming as a way to explore communication, as well as to create interactive characters to express fears and feelings. For example, I conducted a pilot study at Children's Hospital in Boston with young cardiac patients who used SAGE to cope with cardiac illness, hospitalizations, and invasive medical procedures (Bers et al., 1998). The process of content creation through programming in SAGE allowed children to engage in the developmental work of decentering (Piaget, 1962) and in mastering technological competence as they debugged their characters after observing other people's interactions with them.

The following is a log of an interaction between Damian, a 16 year old waiting for a heart transplant, and a rabbit, the best friend of "Mrs. Needle." Both characters, the rabbit and Mrs. Needle, were created by a younger girl who had previously used SAGE while in the hospital preparing for her own surgery. Damian had never met this girl but was interacting with the characters that she had created:

SAGE: Hi, what is your name?

CHILD: Damian.

SAGE: Welcome, Damian. I am Bunny, the best friend of Mrs. Needle. She hides in the computer because she is a little shy. She thinks that all the kids hate her. So she asked me to talk on her behalf. Is that OK with you?

CHILD: Yes.

SAGE: Wonderful, wonderful, Damian! Mrs. Needle is worried because kids scream when they see her. But, have you met Mrs. Needle before?

CHILD: I guess yes.

SAGE: Well, Mrs. Needle is my best friend and she hides in the computer. Tell me, Damian, how old are you?

CHILD: 16.

SAGE: Wauh, Damian, you are older than me. I wonder if you are as scared of needles as I am? I hate them, all except my friend Mrs. Needle. What about you?

CHILD: They are all right.

SAGE: As I was telling you, Damian, I am Mrs. Needle's best friend and she asked me to find out why children hate her so much. She thinks that it is because she stings, but she is not sure. What do you think?

CHILD: Yes, no kid is excited to get any needles.

SAGE: I see Damian... what else can you tell me about this?

CHILD: The kids are afraid of it because it hurts and they don't like it to hurt and I guess that is it.

SAGE: Guess what, Damian? Mrs. Needle has a story for you. She is shy but she loves to tell stories. She always says that they have power.... Listen to her....

MRS. NEEDLE: They built me to sting, but that is not all I do. If you were a flower I could water you without hurting you. But you are not, and I am not a water pot. My nose is like a hose or like a straw and my belly has goodies than can help you to heal. When my belly is empty, the goodies are yours and you can feel better. But sometimes it is the other way around. My belly starts completely empty, and then it becomes full with your goodies. You can think of me as a someone that only stings, but I also do good. The problem is that this is not always immediately obvious.

SAGE: I loved Mrs. Needle's story, but how about you? Does it somehow relate to what you told me before, Damian?

CHILD: Yes it does.

SAGE: I see, Damian, please explain to me the connection. I don't get it.

CHILD: The children don't realize that the stuff can help them, the medicine.

SAGE: I see, Damian, you got the power of the story. I am sure my friend Mrs. Needle will be very happy. I wish that you will always have the courage to keep telling and listening to stories. I hope to see you soon.... Bye!

After playing with "Mrs. Needle," Damian decided to create his own character called "Mr. Tape." He created the conversational structure, the scripts that "Mr. Tape" says, and also the stories that he tells. Afterward, he interacted with the character and invited other people in the Cardiac Unit to play with it. The following is a saved computer log of Damian's interaction:

SAGE: Hi my name is Mr. Tape. What is yours?

CHILD: Damian.

SAGE: Well hello, Damian, my name is Mr. Tape. I am very sticky, as you probably may know; a lot of children don't like tape because when you have to take it off it hurts. Some kids like to put me anywhere, like the face, hands, just for fun. Do you like tape?

CHILD: No.

SAGE: I am sorry, why don't you like me? Does it hurt you?

CHILD: Sometimes, yes.

SAGE: Well, I am good for taping things up that are broken and I come in different kinds. I try to do the best I can with making things back to normal. So, Damian, how old are you?

CHILD: 16.

SAGE: You are lucky to be able to live that long. My life expectancy is only two to three years. Some people use me up fast and sometimes I am forgotten in the junk drawer. I get pretty lonely in there. Would you like to hear my story?

CHILD: Yes.

SAGE: When I am used as medical tape I am number one for nurses and doctors. I go on IVs and wrap things up. I am good to write on for the nurses to put on IV medication. You can use me for just about everything in the hospital but I am not very sticky for heavier objects. I could be colored on and used for decorations for kids that are very bored. Some people just throw me around and drop me which hurts my feelings, I can't pick them up and drop them, but I thank them for picking me as their number one choice. Well it was nice talking to you, maybe you will talk to me again and listen to my story.

Developing SAGE was my attempt at introducing a new kind of programming language for children in the technological landscape: a language that could allow them to express and explore issues of identity using a narrative metaphor. I strongly believe that we need more of these kinds of environments.

While the constructionist tradition puts programming at the center of children's content creation, a different group of researchers and practitioners, also concerned with providing opportunities for children to create content, focuses on new digital literacies (Buckingham, 2003; Buckingham & Willett, 2006; Coiro, Knobel, Lankshear, & Leu, 2008). This approach is an extension of the media literacy work started in the United States in the early 20th century with the study of film as an active process of consumption, rather than a passive one (National Association for Media Literacy Education, 2009).

Scholars on new digital literacies suggest that with the advances of social media applications, knowledge of computer programming is no longer necessary. Youth can engage in other forms of content creation practices such as instant messaging, blogging, making a Web site, creating and sharing music videos, podcasting and videocasting, working with images and photo sharing, participating in online discussions, e-mailing and using online chat, creating and sharing digital mashups, etc. (see Black, 2008; Coiro, 2003; Gee, 2007; Jenkins, 2006; Kist, 2007; Lankshear & Knobel, 2006; Leu, Kinzer, Coiro, & Cammack, 2004).

Within the digital literacies approach, some work focuses on examining the cognitive and decoding processes involved in comprehending digital texts (Coiro, 2003; Leu, 2001; Leu et al., 2004). Interventions within this approach help children to develop competence in locating, organizing, understanding, evaluating, and analyzing information using digital technology to communicate more efficiently, to verify credible sources online, and to prevent plagiarism (Aviram & Eshet-Alkalai, 2006; Ba, Tally, & Tsikalas, 2002; Eshet-Alkalai, 2004; Eshet-Alkalai & Chajut, 2009; Karlström, Cerratto-Pargman, & Knutsson, 2008; Marsh & Hallet, 2008; McMillan, 1996).

Other work looks at the highly collaborative, distributed, and participatory social practices around the use of new technologies (Jenkins, 2006; Lankshear & Knobel, 2006). Henry Jenkins, Provost's Professor of Communication, Journalism, and Cinematic Arts at the University of Southern California and an influential scholar on media and popular culture, suggests that the increasing access to the Internet has fostered a participatory culture. This new culture has relatively low barriers to artistic expression and civic engagement, strong support for creating and sharing one's creations, informal mentorship where the most experienced pass along expertise to novices, and the members' belief that their contributions matter. Jenkins observes that the democratic tendency in participatory culture allows for the emergence of new models of production and content creation.

When designing our digital landscape, the PTD framework invites us to choose technologies and processes that support content creation. We learn better by doing, by making, by designing. Our digital landscape should provide opportunities for programming projects and for contributing to the growing online participatory culture. In the process of content creation, children develop technological competence by learning new concepts and skills, but most important, they explore new ways of thinking.

Vignette 1

I LOVE YOU, MOMMY: YOUNG CHILDREN AND DIGITAL ART

By Jeewon Kim

Maria, five years old, St. Louis, Mo.
Maria is a five year old growing up in the suburbs of St. Louis, Missouri, with her mother, father, and newborn brother. This year, Maria began attending a local kindergarten, and though her parents experienced some separation anxiety, Maria has thrived so far with her teacher and peers in her first school environment. From the time she was three, Maria has loved to have tea parties. Her sociodramatic play regularly includes stuffed animal royalty sitting around the table and sharing stories of the latest developments in the kingdom. Maria is, of course, the princess of the kingdom, and her dearest possession, Sweetie Bear, is her prince.

Maria attends an National Association for the Education of Young Children–accredited kindergarten with all of the developmentally appropriate tools situated in their respective stations. Her days consist of a carefully scheduled mix of guided groups and activity and open-ended "Choice" time, with small activities accompanied by scaffolding from the head teacher and teaching assistants. Her favorite activities include block play, sand and water tables, finger painting, and of course, tea parties.

Above all, Maria loves to create art on the computer. Her kindergarten offers open-source art software that the children have the opportunity to use in pairs during "Choice" time. The software is multiplatform and features a simple interface geared toward early childhood. A number of drawing tools are provided, including paintbrushes; stamps; text, line, and shape tools; "magic" effects (e.g., blurring, image distortion, color correction); and most important, an eraser. Creations can be saved to a virtual picture book in multiple file formats, including JPEG and PNG.

Maria loves the software so much that her parents downloaded it for their home on her fifth birthday. The software offers Maria an engaging opportunity to participate in content creation. In the process, she learns more about how to use technology. When she first enrolled in the kindergarten, Maria could barely use the mouse and keyboard. Now, she logs in to the software with ease and creates artwork of ever-increasing sophistication. Maria's parents regulate her use of the software at home—art software, like most things, is best in moderation.

The art software most recently brought joy into Maria's life because it enabled her to create customized Christmas cards for each member of her family—her mother, father, baby brother, and even grandmother and grandfather in Florida. Maria's teachers helped her spell her intended holiday greetings with the text tools and printed out her cards at school for her to bring home and surprise her family. Grandma and Grandpa received both a hard copy in the mail and a digital copy via e-mail so that they could forward the cards to other family members and show off Maria's digital prowess. With a simple mouse click, Maria's newfound competence can be shared not only in the classroom, and at home, but with friends and family anywhere in the country.

Vignette 2
LEARNING SCIENCE THROUGH ROBOTICS ENGINEERING

By Amber Kendall

Gabriella, eight years old, Boston, Mass.
Gabriella is a third grader in an urban New England elementary school. Her classroom is participating in a research project using robotics during science lessons. Instead of a traditional science inquiry unit on rocks and minerals, the

class is exploring properties of materials through a grand design problem: building a model house that is sturdy, soundproof, waterproof, and comfortable in all temperatures. As they work on this project over the course of 10 lessons students are gaining experience with technology and engineering, along with science.

The robotics kit they are using, LEGO™ MINDSTORMS, has pieces that are familiar and unfamiliar to Gabriella. When she opens the kit for the first time, she is confronted with not only traditional LEGO pieces, like the bricks, plates, and beams she has at home, but also wheels, gears, axles, and bushings. But when she lifts the top tray of the kit, the newest and most exciting features of all are revealed: the NXT brick, a small, handheld computer, and the motors and sensors it controls. The NXT can be programmed to do many things, including power robots that follow lines on the floor, play music, and draw pictures. In science class, however, the NXT becomes a powerful tool for data collection, allowing the third graders to have access to digital tools that simulate the ones they might use in high school science or even in a research lab. For the unit on properties of materials, Gabriella and her classmates will use the NXT to measure light, sound, and temperature to inform the building of the model house.

The lesson focuses beyond the physical construction of the house. In order to choose the best materials to meet the criteria of "being soundproof, waterproof, and comfortable in all temperatures," Gabriella and her classmates must test materials and make judgments about their suitability. This is where the NXT bricks become important. Gabriella and her partner are given two choices of material for the interior of the house, thin craft foam or cotton batting. In order to test the soundproofing capabilities of these two materials, the pair uses a sound sensor hooked up to the NXT brick. First, as an exploration, the girls are asked to try to find different levels of sound in the classroom. They take turns discovering new areas to test and reading the measurements on the computer screen. Then they get down to the business of testing their materials. A second NXT brick is placed inside a sleeve of the material to be tested, and Gabriella makes that NXT let out a series of beeps as her partner detects the sound level and carefully records each trial in her journal. She shares her data with her partner and then switches roles to test the second material. Gabriella's partner reminds her of the importance of consistency in the experiment to control for variables. Students question or support one another's results while the pros and cons of each material are discussed. When combined with the results from the temperature insulation test, the class decides that craft foam is the best material for achieving the desired sound and thermal insulation goals. While working on this project, Gabriella is developing as a learner, researcher, and team member, not just as a science student.

Vignette 3
DESIGNING A SPACE ON THE WORLD WIDE WEB

By Hera Kan

Sarah, 13 years old, Carson, Calif.
Growing up, Sarah, a 13-year-old girl, never had any creative outlet that she was proud of and never had the confidence to explore different media. Music was not her strong suit, although she tried various instruments from the piano to the violin. She knew she had two left feet, so dancing was out of the question. Drawing and painting? Only if works of art were stick figures and doodles. None of the conventional means for creativity worked for Sarah. She wanted to be an artist who could channel her ideas into a specific medium, but it eluded her.

Finally, it was the summer of 1998, and Sarah's family had finally gained access to high-speed Internet in their home. With the family computer no longer tied to the telephone line, Sarah was able to explore the World Wide Web at her leisure. This was an exciting time for discovery. Having the Internet at home opened so many possibilities, from looking up information for school to finding photos by her favorite photographer.

During her explorations, Sarah began following Web sites of her favorite anime, *Sailor Moon*. She began to realize that these fan sites were made by people just like her, young teenagers and fans. She loved the idea of creating a Web site to connect and share with people who enjoyed the same things as she did. After some initial search, Sarah found some simple tutorials on hypertext markup language (HTML). HTML utilizes paired tags, which a browser reads and then displays as a Web page. Basic HTML allows the ability to add images, color, and video to a Web site.

So Sarah began her journey learning all she could, from embedding images to creating banners that were distinct from everyone else's. Web sites back then were filled with color, music, and moving backgrounds, which would make most people cringe nowadays, but it must be admitted that there was an excitement surrounding them. Sarah dabbled in the craze as well and began to publish sites in her favorite colors and with her favorite content.

As her skills progressed, Sarah became more confident in her ability to learn and create Web sites. The idea of turning simple strings of letters and words into a creative outlet sparked her curiosity. Sarah began to explore the programming. Arriving at the local bookstore, Sarah picked up a C++ primer and hurried home to create her first program, "Hello World."

At this juncture, Sarah became immersed in the idea and concept of programming. Logic and creativity were both required to create a fully functioning program. She began to design simple programs to put on her Web site. One simple program that became a big hit with her circle of friends involved taking a letter a user had written and outputting a "coded" version to send to their friends, who would then have to return to Sarah's site to have the letter decoded.

With this newfound confidence, Sarah began to delve into other forms of creative outlets where she could master a specific technique and apply her own ideas. She began to take classes on computer animation and began to learn photography. As her skill progressed in each of these areas, Sarah would always return to her Web site and display her short animations and photographs. She kept up with the ever-changing HTML code and learned new and various ways to expand her site using Cascading Style Sheets for formatting and appearance and Flash for interactivity. Working on her Web site is Sarah's favored pastime that provides both a challenge and a creative outlet.

CHAPTER 5

Creativity to Build Confidence

The second C, creativity, has a strong relationship with the first one, content creation. Research has shown that, in both sciences and the arts, the most creative innovators also tend to be the most productive (Sawyer, 2006a). A digital landscape that promotes positive development must be a space where children can make projects and develop new skills, a space that supports creative expressions and a strong sense of confidence, a space where new ideas can take on new forms, and a space where traditional approaches can be transcended.

The creativity that the PTD framework advocates for has a "little c," as opposed to Creativity with a "big C." The "little c" creativity includes activities that children engage in every day, for example, using cardboard boxes for making castles, crafting art projects with pencils, dressing up with mom's clothes, writing a poem, or figuring out how to save some extra money for taking a trip with friends. The "big C" Creativity, instead, refers to a field of scientific study that focuses on solving difficult problems in novel and appropriate ways to transform the boundaries of an entire discipline or domain (Sawyer, 2006a). Research in this tradition looks at significant works of geniuses such as Einstein or Mozart or explores how Creativity was defined differently in distinct sociohistorical periods. For example, Keith Sawyer, a professor of psychology and education at Washington University in St. Louis, describes that the idea that an artist creates a novel work that breaks with convention is historically recent. Before the Renaissance, creativity was the ability to imitate the well-established masters and to accurately represent nature (Sawyer, 2006a, chap. 2).

The creative process with a "little c," as we will understand it here, refers to everyone's potential to create and imagine in original ways. However, creativity doesn't just happen. For creativity to flourish there are several requirements: working hard and engaging in a conscious activity that requires training and skills—thus the bidirectional relationship among content creation and mastery, creativity and confidence, and enjoying the process or entering a state of flow (Csikszentmihalyi, 2000). In the creative process, there is never one right answer. There is divergent thinking to generate multiple unique ideas and convergent thinking to combine those ideas into the best result. Contradicting some popular myths on creativity, the creative person is not necessarily the one who wakes up one morning saying, "Eureka!" but, rather, the one who is disciplined in his work and is able to find new connections.

Despite early worries that computers might stifle creativity (Cordes & Miller, 2000; Oppenheimer, 2003), research has found that when used well, open-ended constructionist types of software can actually help creativity to bloom (Clements & Sarama, 2003; Resnick, 2007b). Mitchel Resnick (2006) presents a vision of how children might use computers in a creative way, as if they were paintbrushes to playfully explore, experiment, design, and invent.

Unfortunately our digital landscape is vastly populated by edutainment software that may deprive children of the opportunity to engage in creative projects. Resnick writes:

> They provide entertainment as a reward if you are willing to suffer through a little education. Or they boast that you will have so much fun using their products that you won't even realize that you are learning—as if learning were the most unpleasant experience in the world. . . . Part of the problem is with the word *edutainment* itself. When people think about *education* and *entertainment*, they tend to think of them as services that someone else provides for you. Studios, directors, and actors provide you with entertainment; schools and teachers provide you with education. New edutainment companies try to provide you with both. In all of these cases, you are viewed as a passive recipient. But that's not the way most learning happens. In fact, you are likely to learn the most, and enjoy the most, if you are engaged as an active participant, not a passive recipient. (2006, pp. 3–4)

As previously mentioned, creativity is intimately tied with the possibility of creating projects, the first C of the PTD framework. A creative person in the domain of technology can imagine new ways of expressing her technological competence. She is not afraid of technology; she knows that she has the skills, and if not, she is confident that she has the intellectual tools and resources to acquire them.

Confidence can be defined as the perception that one can achieve desired goals through one's actions. In the technological domain, a confident child is someone who can act successfully, or believes she can learn how to act, in the digital landscape. She can make an interactive birthday card; she can program a computer game, write a blog, create a Web site, or learn how to use a new software package to make 3-D animations. This child has the needed skills to create a project, the ability to find help when necessary, and the perseverance to work hard when faced with technical difficulties. She doesn't give up. She knows she can do it, either by herself or with someone's assistance.

Researchers have found self-efficacy (or self-efficacy beliefs) to be a necessary component for successfully using technologies to complete tasks (Cassidy & Eachus, 2002; Coffin & MacIntyre, 1999). However, confidence is not a single, global concept. Although some children may see themselves as generally confident with technology, others might experience confidence differently when approaching different tasks. For example, one might feel confident when programming in Scratch, while someone else might feel confident working with digital pictures, posting on social networks, or building robots. As with everything else, confidence is expressed differently at different ages. A teenager who hopes to become a software engineer might see himself as someone who knows a lot about computers; a four year old who is learning to navigate the screen interface will be confident in his ability to save and open a file. Both will know that they have the skills needed to achieve the desired goal.

Competence and confidence often go hand in hand: the more competent someone is, the more likely that she will feel confident. In turn, confidence can reinforce competence. Believing that we can succeed allows us to work hard at further developing our skills. Richard Lerner explains this in simple terms: "Competence is about what you can do. Confidence is about how you feel—or rather what you believe you can do. It is a more interior quality. We are confident if we perceive ourselves to be competent" (2007, p. 76).

An important aspect of confidence is the belief that people can improve their skills. The perception of progress is important for trusting in one's potential. It allows us to understand failure as a step toward success. This is at the core of most design-based endeavors that involve working from an initial idea to a finished product. Mitchel Resnick (2007b) refers to this process as a spiraling creative cycle.

As designers inspired by the PTD framework we want to choose digital landscapes that provide multiple opportunities for this type of process: children imagine what they want to do, create a project based on their ideas, play with materials and their creations, share their ideas and creations with others, reflect on their experiences—all of which leads them to imagine new ideas and new projects. The iterative steps of the spiraling creative cycle (imagine, create, play, share, reflect) are similar to those found in the engineering design process mentioned in previous chapters.

However, at the center is imagination, as opposed to finding a solution to a problem. This is a subtle distinction. In the 21st century many of our needs require us not only to engage in problem solving but also to develop creative thinking skills to frame problems in innovative ways both at the micro- and macrolevels (Bronson & Merryman, 2010; Sawyer, 2006b). A technological landscape that supports positive youth development must provide opportunities for children to learn new ways of approaching the unexpected situations that will continually arise in their lives.

All creativity involves the act of creation. However, not all acts of creation involve creativity. The PTD approach suggests that we should design and advocate for digital landscapes that support both content creation and creativity. For example, when a four year old uses Kid Pix to create a story and presents a slideshow to her parents, or when a five year old uses the CHERP programming language to make robots that can dance the hokey pokey and move around in search of food, technology is opening a door to creativity. When a 10 year old combines recyclables and traditional art materials with technological components, or when a 12 year old can take a robotic base and turn it into anything he wants—from a monster truck to a kitty cat, from a flower to an interactive garden—technology is being used in creative ways. One of the potentials of our digital landscape is that it can offer creative technologies that can be programmed to take on a "thousand forms" for a "thousand functions" and appeal to a "thousand tastes" (Papert, 1980).

Vignette 1
THE SIMS

By Ben Peirce

Ben, 13 years old, New Castle, N.H.
Fresh out of seventh grade, Ben is looking forward to a summer of mental relaxation. After months of homework, quizzes, and the occasional all-nighter, he is ready to lose himself to sleep, television, and general inactivity. However, his vacation will not be as devoid of stimulation as he might have thought, thanks to a newly released computer game called The Sims. This is the summer Ben became an architect.

Ben has just finished his latest project: a two-story, four-bedroom house for the newest members of his virtual neighborhood. Over the past two hours, he has poured over dozens of possible physical features, outfits, and personality traits to assign to each of his newly created denizens; he feels that each member should be unique in appearance and attitudes yet compatible with the rest of the family (they will, after all, be sharing a home). Once he is satisfied with his choices, he dubs his latest family "the Oddballs" and selects an empty lot to build upon. While he is technically free to use any materials he sees fit to construct this new house, he is limited by a fixed budget of digital seed money; he cannot expect to see a cash influx until the Oddballs start their job hunts (another process he will have to plan out carefully). Thus, for the time being, he builds a simple structure: four walls, two floors, eight rooms, 16 windows, one roof, and one front door. Now it is time to go shopping.

Using the remainder of his initial budget, he purchases cheap but reliable furniture and appliances for the Oddballs. In the end he has a living room (comprising a couch and a small TV), kitchen (with a fridge, stove, and dining table), bathroom (consisting of one shower, toilet, and sink), four upstairs bedrooms (each consisting of a small twin bed and a nightstand), and one empty space. As soon as the Oddballs can learn to support themselves and save a little extra cash, he plans to buy them more sources of entertainment as a reward for their hard work. Besides, they will need more exciting wares than this to attract the attention of the other virtual families living up and down the street. Once the Oddballs begin to interact with their neighbors, Ben will choose to either let their relationships take their own courses or guide them as he sees fit. For in the town of Simville, Ben isn't just the mayor: he is God.

The Sims is a computer game that allows users like Ben to build their own communities of virtually controlled inhabitants. The program encourages creativity in that it prompts players to find their own unique solutions to a myriad of logistical problems: What should an "ideal" house look like? How can one make the most of limited funds? What is the best way to obtain more resources? When is a good time to expand/renovate?

Answers do not present themselves readily. Given the excess of freedom and control, it is not uncommon for players to build themselves into corners. Users might spend too much money erecting walls and not enough feeding their characters; they could construct a beautiful kitchen only to watch it burn when a cheap appliance malfunctions and starts a fire; or they can fail to provide their inhabitants with necessities or enough stimulation, leaving them bored and unhappy. But through trial and error they can seek a balance between efficiency and ingenuity, resulting in better houses and happier characters. Once Ben attains a more complete understanding of the game's rules, he will no longer have to rely on the trial-and-error method and will anticipate possible outcomes before they occur, leading to more successful projects in less time. He will learn new skills as he goes from constructing simple shacks with lazy roommates to maintaining sprawling mansions that house productive and interesting members of the community.

Also, while this program does not allow him to interact or communicate with other players over the Internet, it does have the potential to let him role-play. Because he can control the actions of his characters, he can choose to make them act civilly or disrespectfully toward each other. But although he can manage their physical actions, Ben cannot manually manipulate their emotions. Every character interaction prompts the virtual participants to feel a specific emotion that is out of Ben's control. Thus, Ben can experiment with a number of different personalities and behaviors in a risk-free environment and explore what kinds of interactions yield positive results.

Vignette 2
EXPANDING HUMAN CAPACITIES

By Kenneth Tae-Han Lee

Ken, 18 years old, Fullerton, Calif.

Music was Ken's life. For every waking moment, Ken always had a song in his head. During school exams, social gatherings with friends, golf and tennis tournaments, or even religious services, Ken's mind was a radio station running without advertisements—to the point where he walked the thin line of being either a music fanatic, which interfered with his social well-being, or an avid music listener. He was so infatuated with music that after hearing the first 15 seconds of any song on the radio, he could identify the song's title and artist. Ken would then be able to recite the chorus of that song within the next 10 seconds.

However, Ken's love for music did not translate into being a musician. Not only was he tone deaf and unable to sing a note, but he also lacked any sort of virtuosity in playing an instrument. Try as he might, no amount of practice, lessons, or passion would make his fingers dance on top of the 88 keys on a piano, slide along the neck of a guitar or bass, or orient themselves in the right placement and location on any woodwind or brass instrument. To make matters even worse, he lacked any and all forms of rhythm. Attempting to play the drums resulted in such a cacophony that Ken was partially convinced that he could start an exterminator business by playing the drums to scare off rodents and termites from ever entering the house again.

A culmination of multiple failures in attempting to play an instrument led to such a depleted feeling of self-worth that Ken had given up his dream of becoming a musician. However, he found a small sliver of hope when he was introduced to the DJ world at the age of 18. DJ-ing involves transitioning from one song to another in order to produce a continuous flow of music. This is usually performed at parties where attendees dance incessantly for hours. Because being a DJ fit Ken's profile better than playing an instrument, Ken took the plunge and decided to take one more shot at being a musician.

Initially, DJ-ing was a success compared with Ken's previous attempts at learning an instrument. Ken's vast knowledge of music induced some form of progress—after a week, he was able to perform the rudimentary steps of DJ-ing such as selecting popular songs that party attendees would enjoy and finding ways to creatively transition between them. However, after three months' worth of practice, blistered fingers, and ringing eardrums, the endeavor seemed fruitless. Inevitably, Ken's lack of musical talent finally caught up to him, as he saw no improvement in his skill set as a DJ. Since DJ-ing was Ken's last shot at being a musician, he looked toward technology as his last stand or "Hail Mary." Unknowingly, Ken stumbled upon technology that would change his capacity as a DJ.

Recent technological innovations in DJ-ing have produced computer software that plays music and provides the pitch and tempo of each song. More important, this software creates visualizations of the wavelengths of each song. With this visualization, Ken was able to see the points where the music would be at a higher or lower volume, as well as the chorus or main points of the song. After buying this technology and practicing with it for an hour, Ken saw vast improvements in his skill set. It was as if he was given a cheat sheet to DJ-ing. His computer program instantly did most of what Ken was trying to do on his own accord. This technology drastically extended Ken's human capacities and musical talent. For Ken, DJ-ing changed from a difficult and seemingly futile endeavor to an exciting and gratifying experience.

This increase in Ken's skill led to him being hired for events and parties, which in turn led to an upward spike in his confidence and feeling of self-worth. Jutting out his chest, Ken would proudly show his face during his events and started developing a style that became synonymous with his pseudonym, DJ KEN-EKT. Whereas Ken's first gigs consisted of him playing the most popular songs on the radio, he gradually improved as a DJ and began to tell stories with his performances. At one of his performances, Ken selected and transitioned between songs that centered on finding one's first true love; at another performance, he induced the message of forgetting the past and focusing on the sanctity of the present and future. Steadily, Ken began performing at increasingly larger venues. As DJ KEN-EKT became somewhat of a faux celebrity, he attracted the attention of two other local DJs who offered him a proposition that he could not refuse—to form an enterprise revolving around DJ-ing services.

As a result, Ken became one of the cofounders of L.R.G. Entertainment, a small, albeit steady business that helped him reach his dream of being a musician. And to think, Ken would never have fulfilled his dream if it were not for technology.

Vignette 3
THE 10 PLAGUES

By Tali Bers

Tali, 10 years old, Arlington, Mass.
Tali goes to a Jewish day school in the Boston area that embraces a wide range of Jewish expression, practice, and belief. Tali plays the piano and likes to hang out with her friends. She has two younger brothers.

At school Tali is learning about the book of Exodus, which tells the story of the departure of the Israelites from Egypt, which marked the end of a period of oppression for Abraham's descendants who were slaves in Egypt, and the journey led by Moses into the Promised Land. In class, the teacher usually asks students to make a drawing to show their learning or to write a story. But this time, there was a special surprise. They were going to use computers.

Each child was asked to think about a particular aspect of the story he or she was most interested in. They were then invited to create an animation using Scratch. Tali chose to do the 10 plagues. When Moses asked Pharaoh to let his people go, to free them from slavery in Egypt, he was given no as an answer. The story says that God sent the plagues to soften Pharaoh's heart. Tali was fascinated by the plagues. She wanted to know what they meant. For example, she thought how terrible it must have been for the Egyptians when the water turned into blood. She imagined that back then there were no faucets or bottled water, and people and animals needed the river to drink. Tali also thought about the plague of darkness that turned Egypt all dark. She got scared, as she knew that they did not have electricity or candles, so they needed the sun, the moon, and the stars.

She wondered what the plagues would be now. She imagined what would make her really scared. She decided to create a Scratch project to show the plagues then and now. She referred back to the Exodus story to create the "then" animation, and she used her imagination to create the "now" animation. Tali was very excited about her idea and worked hard. First, she had to remember all the plagues. She opened her book and read the passages that talked about the plagues. She also went online to search for pictures that could represent each plague. For each plague that happened in Egypt, she imagined an equivalent one that would happen now.

For example, she read about the frogs that jumped all over Egypt scaring people, and she thought about the recent earthquake in Haiti. She decided that earthquakes were one of the plagues of today's world. Using the drawing tool in Scratch she created a picture of an earthquake. She recorded herself saying,

"Bam, bam, bam sh shsh." Then she read about how the locusts ate all the crops in Egypt and that led to starvation, and she thought that if all the cows died, we might not have any more meat today. So she created an animation of animals dying and recorded sound. For the last and most terrible plague, the death of each firstborn Egyptian boy, she thought about global warming. Tali is really concerned about global warming; she learned about it listening to the radio while her mom drives her to school. She drew a picture of the world, animated it to change colors, and drew shining fire on it. Tali had learned that the Exodus story says that God had sent the plagues to Egypt, but she believes that today people are creating their own plagues, for example, global warming, by not taking care of the planet.

Tali was proud of her final project. She worked hard to create the "then" and "now" of the 10 plagues. She used both knowledge about the biblical story and creativity to imagine what could happen today. During the final presentation, parents were invited to see the Scratch projects. Tali was very proud. A few projects were picked to show at a technology fair for local schools. Tali's was one of them. She and three of her friends got to show off their projects, answer questions from visitors, and see projects from other schools. Tali felt very pleased with herself and confident about her technological abilities. She is hoping to work with Scratch again next year.

CHAPTER 6

Choices of Conduct to Develop Character Traits

A digital landscape that affords opportunities for content creation and creativity, the previously explored C's, while helpful for developing technological expertise, is not enough for orienting youth regarding how and when to use those skills. This chapter focuses on the third C, choices of conduct. It advances the notion that programming languages, virtual worlds, and social media, among other technologies, can become ethical playgrounds to explore our moral identities.

The digital landscape, like the playground, must allow the freedom for children to make authentic choices, to experience consequences, to take risks, and to reflect on their actions. Of course there is the safety issue. The kinds of fences we build around the playground and the degrees of freedom of exploration will be determined by the age of the child and her developmental needs, as well as the comfort zone of the adult in charge.

The process of making choices is an important aspect of building a strong sense of character. Character is not simply about how we feel or think but also about the actions we take. It is about having a moral purpose, a sense of responsibility and moral commitment, not only for our own self-growth but for the improvement of society (Colby & Damon, 1992; Damon, 1990). Our choices should not violate the social contract and should support society and its institutions, social justice, and a sense of fairness. Richard Lerner summarizes this idea: "There is a delicate balance between serving oneself and acting selflessly for the good of other individuals or society" (2007, p. 139). When designing our digital landscape, the PTD framework reminds us that we must provide opportunities for children to evolve an internal moral compass to guide their actions in the world.

This perspective is strongly influenced by Piaget's belief that moral development emerges from action; that is to say, individuals construct their knowledge about morality as a result of interactions with the environment and experiences rather than pure imitation (Piaget, 1965). In other words, morality is not learned by simply internalizing the norms of a group but, rather, by a developmental process that involves personal struggles to arrive at fair solutions. Extending Piaget's work on moral judgment in the child, Lawrence Kohlberg (1973) understood moral development as an increasing ability to perceive and integrate social experience through taking diverse roles. Robert Selman (2003) has further advanced this work by focusing on perspective taking and perspective coordination, the ability to coordinate one's own point of view with others' viewpoints in social interactions and relationships.

Kohlberg identified six stages of moral development. These start with value judgments of a highly egocentric form (i.e., "What I like is what is good"), followed by a decentering process (i.e., "Something is good because it is good for somebody else"). The final stage is reached when abstract moral principles develop (i.e., "I don't kill because killing is bad" [Kohlberg, 1976]). The assumption behind this approach, as well as that of Piaget, is that there is a universal progression from concrete to abstract ways of thinking about moral issues. For example, Kohlberg understands "justice" as the key concept that an individual develops when engaging in higher stages of moral judgment. In his view, progression happens as a result of moral reasoning. Carol Gilligan (1982) complemented this work by focusing on how women construct the moral domain and how they approach and resolve dilemmas in a different way than men. Critiques of the idea that the highest stage of development involves abstraction and logical reasoning propose the need for and validity of different thinking styles (Papert, 1987; Turkle & Papert, 1992).

Methodologically speaking, Kohlberg used hypothetical moral dilemmas to study and promote moral reasoning ability (Blatt & Kohlberg, 1975). He emphasized reflection and discussion about the dilemmas, but the moral decisions themselves were not of primary importance; rather, it was the reasoning that was used to arrive at the decisions. Although Kohlberg is most well known for his stages of moral development, much of the unexplored promise of his work lies in the "just community" model (Kohlberg, 1985; Reed, 1997). This approach proposes that involvement in participatory democracy, social institutions, group decision making, and self-government is critical in shaping the individual's moral development. Reasoning is not enough. Moral lives, and not only moral thinking, are needed.

In 2008, the Josephson Institute's Center for Youth Ethics conducted a nationwide survey of nearly 30,000 American high school students. The study found "entrenched habits of dishonesty—stealing, lying, and cheating." Moreover, despite their own responses detailing their dishonest habits, 93% of students said that they "were satisfied with their personal ethics and character" (Josephson Institute of Ethics, 2008). We live in a difficult, contradictory, and ambiguous world where the "right decisions" are often difficult to make.

Digital landscapes can provide opportunities for young people to explore their moral identities. This need has served as my guiding compass through all my own work, from robotics to virtual worlds and from programming languages to storytelling environment. For example, the Zora virtual world has built-in mechanisms to create a Kholbergian "just community," a safe space to experiment with ways of thinking and behaving needed to function in a community, but also a space to test personal and moral values through actions and conversations. Another example, the SAGE programming environment, encourages children to think about their most cherished role models and their inspirations. The database of stories offered by the wise storytellers is organized around values. The robotics projects that I have implemented in Jewish day schools in the United States, the Mi Ani project (Libman, 2011), and the Con-ciencia project in Argentina (Bers & Urrea, 2000) invite children to create robots to represent cherished values. Regardless of the choice of technology, the focus on moral identity is always present in my work.

Let me tell you a story of what happened during one of the first studies that I conducted with Zora in 1999 with a multicultural group of teenagers participating in an intensive three-week Zora workshop at the MIT Media Lab (Bers, 2001). During the second day of the workshop, children discovered the need to create laws to make living in the virtual world easier. This realization happened as they started to play with Zora to test its technical limitations. For example, they created huge virtual objects and left them in inadequate virtual places, and they learned how to distort the look of personal avatars and how to change the size of other people's virtual homes. Although they were developing competence and confidence regarding the technology, they were not wise in their choices for using their expertise. At the beginning it was fun, but soon it became hard to "live" that way. Children were getting upset as their creations were modified without permission, and the virtual world was becoming messy and disorganized.

The idea of laws for self-organization emerged in a natural way, as a need of the community and not as a suggestion from an external agent, such as a teacher or facilitator, or as a limitation of the technology (i.e., it was my design decision to potentially allow for these things to happen, as opposed to implementing a permissions system in Zora to prevent potential chaos). In the first City Hall virtual meeting, children elected a city mayor and asked him to coordinate a discussion about rules for Zora. After a long debate, the children agreed on some basic rules:

> No putting things in people's personal rooms, no warping [modifying] people or their things, set the properties of the objects placed in public spaces so others can clone them, people can make their own rules for their own rooms but it must be clear, the junk room can never be too full, fess up to what you do and there will be no jail.

During the following days kids continued meeting in the virtual City Hall. For example, one day there was a heated discussion about "punishment" for those who intentionally broke some of the rules. Nino, a 14-year-old boy, advocated for locking people up in a virtual jail, while others proposed virtual community service as a form of punishment. The children spent a considerable amount of online time discussing how to technically implement a virtual jail so avatars couldn't escape. They were aware that choices needed to be informed by competent knowledge. The children considered the possibility of electing someone to be "prison guard," but no one wanted that role because "it is too boring to always stay in the same place and go after people." Finally, they reached a consensus and created a new law: "Punishment for breaking a rule is to write a positive value in the Zora dictionary."

The possibility of choosing our actions and accepting their consequences, as opposed to following prescribed rules, is an important aspect of moral development. Children need to experiment with "what if" situations and examine their values and ethical choices. These experiences help them develop character traits that will serve them well in leading moral lives. In turn, their evolving moral compass will guide their choices of conduct. Thus, in the PTD framework, the pair choices of conduct/character traits plays an important role. As we will see later, it has a strong relationship with the pair community building/contribution.

Although most of these explorations naturally happen online, the technological landscape offers many opportunities to design experiences to promote choices of conduct and community building. In my work with robotics and kindergartners, I am aware of this (Bers, 2008a). For example, most robotic programs in educational settings give each group of children an already sorted kit with all the needed materials to build a robot. In my work with the TangibleK program we take a different approach (Bers, 2010b). We sort all materials by types and place them in bins in the center of the room (instead of giving an already sorted robotic kit to each child or group). Children learn how to take what they need without depleting the bins of the "most wanted" pieces, such as special sensors or colorful minifigures. They also learn how to negotiate for what they need. The TangibleK program, inspired by the PTD philosophy, focuses not only on learning about robotics but also on helping young children develop an inner compass to guide their actions in a just and responsible way (Bers, 2010b).

The nature of social media and social gaming extends the possibility for young people to engage in decision making, perspective taking, conflict resolution, and values clarification. These are all aspects of moral development. Howard Gardner's GoodPlay Project explores some of these various ethical dimensions in the digital media experiences of today's youth (James et al., 2009). The 2008 Pew Internet and American Life Project's report found that 44% of youth play games that teach them about a problem in society, while 52% play games that cause them to think about moral and ethical issues (Lenhart et al., 2008). The report also suggests that youth with civic gaming experiences are more likely to be civically engaged in the offline world by getting information online, persuading others regarding voting in elections, and raising money for charity. Kahne, Middaugh, and Evans (2008) found that "the stereotype of the antisocial game" was not reflected in the data from their study, as "youth who play games frequently are just as civically and politically active as those who play games infrequently" (p. 27).

Researchers such as Williams (2006b) suggest that the backdrop for the rise of social gaming is a decline in civic shared spaces for people to meet and converse face-to-face. Echoing Oldenburg's (1997) account of how third places—which are neither home nor work and cross-nationally might include social clubs, *tabernas*, piazzas, pubs, and public squares—are vital for community formation and maintenance, some researchers suggest that virtual multiplayer games might fulfill the need for community and social interaction (Steinkuehler, 2006). For example, the virtual world Quest Atlantis, developed by Sasha Barab and his team at Indiana University, embeds civic learning opportunities in the quest for students to find solutions to the problems faced by a fictional world called Atlantis (Barab et al., 2005).

Levine and Lopez (2002) cite political blogs, "boycott" movements, and transnational youth networks facilitated by new technologies as new venues and opportunities for youth to engage and lead. Yet they contend that amid all these new activities, many young people still lack the skills and "know-how" to carry debates and dialogues beyond their social networks to participate in politics and address public problems. The last chapter of this part of the book, which focuses on community building and contribution, will expand on this.

Vignette 1
HIGH SCHOOL STUDENTS AND VIDEO GAMES

By Amber Kendall

Patrick, 17 years old, and James, 16 years old, Raleigh, N.C.
Patrick received his first video game system, an original PlayStation, for his fourth birthday. His family was not new to video games, as his parents had grown up with arcades and playing Atari and his brother, James, with Nintendo and various computer games. Both Patrick and James have played video games for most of their childhood and consider it one of their chief hobbies; when they are not at school or working, they can most likely be found, each in his own room, playing games in front of the TV or computer.

Patrick received an Xbox 360 for Christmas when he was 14. With it, he also received a subscription to the online gaming service Xbox LIVE so that he could connect to game servers and play online. While the rest of his family is used to a culture where video games are played in isolation, or perhaps with one other person, most of the games popular now, through computers and systems such as the Xbox 360 and Nintendo Wii, offer an instant online connection to players down the street or throughout the world. Unlike his brother, who games for the story or for level mastery and resource management, Patrick plays to interact with people. Through a microphone headset, Patrick is able to talk to the other players, formulating strategies and trash-talking to opponents.

This level of communication while gaming is unprecedented in previous generations. Sometimes Patrick starts games with people he knows from school or from summer camp, and sometimes the games include complete strangers from anywhere across the globe. If he enjoys playing with a new person, he can add that player as a friend and preferentially join his or her games when they are both online.

James, on the other hand, likes to play strategy-based games. He sometimes connects online to play, but unlike Patrick, he prefers plot and character development to competition and collaboration. One fantasy role-playing game James plays on his computer, World of Warcraft, has a huge online following, and players must join factions and build specialized characters. Unlike Patrick's choices for characters in war simulations, James develops his characters from Level 1 and tailors them to function as a team with other specialized players.

These fantasy role-playing games provide many paths players can take to accomplish quests, not simply the "capture-the-flag" mentality of Patrick's favorite games. In James's games, if you make a decision that angers other players or nonplayer characters, that choice may affect later plot elements and interactions with people or open new plot lines and cut others off completely. These choices of conduct are quantified in many games as alignment or karma and become as important an aspect of your character as how fast or strong you are. James's in-game decisions determine how the story will end, and he will often play through a game a second time, making different decisions at pivotal points, to experience new outcomes. Even in games where the player portrays a character who exists in opposition to the law, such as the popular Grand Theft Auto games, players are given a choice in their actions that may reflect their own moral code in the given situation.

Patrick explores choices of conduct a little differently. Since his online gaming is generally team-vs.-team-style combat, absent of moral choices beyond beating the opposing team, his character choices must result instead from how he interacts socially with other people playing the game. The Xbox LIVE servers are monitored to remove any user names or personal information that may be considered offensive, and the censors are very strict—they kick players off the service for repeat offenses. The audio pathways players use to communicate with their headsets during the game, however, are unmonitored. Because expletives are not generally banned in Patrick's house, he can be heard using them during particularly hard matches. A fair number of benign insults are traded between teams, but racial slurs and other more offensive attacks are not uncommon. Patrick is held to whatever standard his parents enforce while they are within earshot, but the choice is his whether to engage in or ignore banter initiated by other players. The decision lies largely in his fellow players. When playing with friends, insults are generally no more derogatory than would be found on the basketball court or in the cafeteria at school; when playing with strangers, particularly those older than he, the urge to fit in socially may override Patrick's default mode of conduct.

Vignette 2
CLEANING UP AFTER THE "TROLLS"

By Jeewon Kim

Christian, 14 years old, Amarillo, Tex.
Christian is a 14-year-old high school sophomore from Amarillo, a city in the north part of Texas near the Oklahoma border. Christian is a freshman at his local public high school and has unfortunately had some difficulties transitioning into his new school environment. A dominant class hierarchy rules the school, and Christian's freshman status puts him at the bottom of the totem pole. Nevertheless, Christian has managed to carve out a niche for himself. While he'll never be a top pick for dodge ball in gym class, or a sought-after date for the Homecoming dance, Christian is a dedicated and respected member of his school's Otaku club. *Otaku* refers to an individual with a strong interest in Japanese anime (cartoons) and/or manga (comic books) and, to a lesser extent, Japanese culture in general. Otaku is somewhat parallel to the more familiar idea of a Trekkie in American culture.

Christian attends the Otaku club every week, where showings of anime are presented and manga are traded and discussed. The students also sample

Japanese food and drink at their after-school meetings. Christian gained popularity quickly in the club because of his vast knowledge of manga and his many limited-edition comics that he shares with the group. Christian's *otaku* interests extend into the digital world as well. At age 14, he serves as the moderator of the forum of a popular Japanese video game franchise. A forum, or message board, is essentially an online discussion site or the digital equivalent of a bulletin board. Members of a forum typically share a common interest and exchange thoughts, ideas, and other user-generated content regarding the topic at hand.

This particular forum is intended for fans of the Legend of Zelda, a popular Nintendo video game franchise. The series has spawned numerous games dating back to the early 1990s, with new installments created for each modern video game platform. In addition, manga and anime have been created starring the characters from the series and serving to expand the mythology of the Zelda universe. The moderator of a forum serves in an administrative role—maintaining the appearance of the forum and more important, the content. Christian's forum is popular, in part, because it adheres to a strict content maintenance policy. Appropriate content includes any and all discussion of the Legend of Zelda franchise (e.g., tips and hints for the video games, favorite characters, upcoming releases, etc.) and also the sharing of fan fiction. *Fan fiction* involves short stories written by fans of fictional universes such as that in the Legend of Zelda. Authors imagine the story of what happens to the characters of a universe outside of their respective video game, anime, manga, or otherwise.

Every day, Christian reads the postings of his digital peers and contributes his own. He also spends time defending his forum from the onslaught of digital bullies, or "trolls," who "flame" and "spam" his message board. "Flaming" consists of vulgar, angry content, usually directed at individual forum users and often containing racist or homophobic slurs. "Spamming" consists of multiple messages meant to clog a forum and annoy its users. "Trolls" are the individuals who conduct this poor behavior, for little more reason than the fun associated with bothering others. Adolescent boys are often characterized by their immature natures, but at 14, Christian is nothing of the sort. While "trolls," most likely near his age range, pollute the digital atmosphere, Christian cleans up their wrongdoing and, with a "three strikes and you're out" policy, sometimes even barring certain users from participation in his forum. Christian's role as a moderator exemplifies the choices of conduct to engage in ethically and morally responsible actions guided by the development of positive character traits.

Christian's story identifies the positive potential of digital entertainment like video games that is little discussed by the media, which is in favor of scare tactics with new items tying video games to physical violence (especially school shootings). While the dangerous potential of video games must be addressed, few things come without both risks and rewards. To acknowledge both the potentially negative and positive outcomes of a digital medium is to authentically evaluate it.

Vignette 3
A DIGITAL RITE OF PASSAGE

By Amanda Sullivan

Laura, 17 years old, Kirkland, Wa.

Laura is a 17-year-old girl and a senior in high school from Kirkland, Washington. Like most teens, Laura has a Facebook profile page that she enjoys maintaining and using to socialize with her friends and classmates. Facebook is a popular social networking Web site that allows users to create and update a personal profile online. A typical profile page includes a photo, a "wall" where other users can post comments, a list of friends with links to their profiles, and a written self-description. Laura's favorite activity on Facebook is editing her profile picture and creating photo albums of her and her friends. In fact, she posts just about every picture she takes, no matter how silly or ridiculous, on Facebook. Laura and her friends post written messages regularly on each other's walls too, sharing gossip on everything from boyfriends and parties to teachers and classmates.

Until recently, Laura had never given a second thought to her choices of conduct on- or offline. But like millions of teenagers, Laura recently faced a huge problem: her mom had friend-requested her on Facebook. At the time, Laura's mind (understandably panicked) flooded with a million questions as she stared in disbelief at the screen: *What will my mom see if I accept her friend request? What can she see even if I don't accept her friend request? What do I want people (like my mom) to think of me based on my Facebook profile page?* Laura realized that she couldn't answer any of these questions easily. Clicking through the Web site, she was disturbed to realize that she had a very limited understanding of Facebook's privacy settings and policies. Laura realized she had never given her online self-presentation the attention it deserved before this moment.

Through reading the Web site's privacy policy, Laura was surprised to learn how many people could see the pictures and comments she and her friends were posting. Feeling uneasy about many of her photos, she was relieved to learn that there were easy ways to limit who sees what content on her profile page. This got Laura thinking: just like offline, there are some behaviors that are only appropriate in *some* settings, some that are appropriate in *all* settings, and some that are simply *never* appropriate. With this in mind, Laura tailored the settings of her profile so that things that were only meant for her closest friends stayed that way. Certain pictures, videos, and public gossip that were deemed never appropriate, Laura got rid of completely.

Ever since Laura officially became "friends" with her mom on Facebook, she has been more cognizant of her conduct both on- and offline. In talking to her older brother James, she began to think of cleaning up her online act as a rite of passage into adulthood. James informed her that when he was a senior in high school and applying to colleges, he went through the same Facebook grooming process. Now excited, Laura spent hours looking through all of her photos and videos and asked herself: *Is this something I want college admissions officers to see? Is this something I want potential employers to see? Am I this person?* If the answer was no, she deleted the content.

Using Facebook's privacy controls and going through an online grooming and purging process made Laura feel like an adult. She continues to use Facebook to interact with her friends, but in a much more responsible way. (And yes, she now happily uses Facebook to socialize with her mom too!)

CHAPTER 7

Communication for Promoting Connections

This chapter is the first of three focused on the possibilities for interpersonal experiences facilitated by the digital landscape. To relate to others, we need to communicate with them. Communication is a process by which meaning is assigned and conveyed in an attempt to create shared understanding. The PTD approach advocates for a technological landscape that supports different forms of communication (e.g., text, voice, sound, pictures, and videos) through synchronous and asynchronous mechanisms to promote positive youth development. Although communication in the online world and social media applications involves some risks, programs informed by PTD must welcome the enormous possibilities for sharing ideas, thoughts, and feelings, for forming new social relationships and maintaining old ones, offered by our technological landscape.

Although sometimes the term *communication* is defined as an "exchange of data and information," within the PTD framework the focus is on communication to promote connection between peers or between youngsters and adults. The question is, "How are the communication mechanisms of the technological landscape supporting the formation and sustainment of positive connections?"

In 1949, when working for Bell Laboratories, Claude Shannon and Warren Weaver developed the first quantifiable theory of communication by using a mathematical model to represent the information flow between sender and receiver, through a channel, and the interference or noise that causes communication to break. This model, often referred to as the transmission model, simply views communication as a means of sending and receiving information. Norbert Wiener (1948), founding father of the discipline of cybernetics, the interdisciplinary study of the structure of physical and social regulatory systems, extended this approach to communication by focusing on the feedback loop that affects the system. Understanding communication as a nonlinear system was a major breakthrough from the linear transmission model, which focused on "who says what to whom in what channel with what effect."

As humans we are meaning-making individuals. We cannot think about communication without thinking about interpretation. When communicating, people might have different purposes, unequal power relations, diverse situational contexts, and different cultural backgrounds and psychological characteristics that influence the process of communication. Communication stands so deeply rooted in human behaviors and the structures of society that to understand it, we need to take all of these factors into consideration. Over the years, Shannon and Weaver's original linear model of communication was expanded to encompass social interaction and interpretation, critical theory and sociocultural approaches, and linguistics and semiotics (Ford, 1994; Piscitelli, 2002).

In the mid-1960s Marshall McLuhan (1964) popularized the idea that "the medium is the message" and proposed that the channel, and not the content it carries or the way the sender and receiver interpret it or the system itself, should be the focus of study. Although controversial, McLuhan's insight was that the characteristics of the medium matter. This has strong implications for thinking about the role of our technological landscape for promoting communication. All technological platforms that support communication are not the same. Each one should be looked at individually, as it might promote or hinder different aspects of connection given the context of its use and the social system it is embedded in. E-mail, video, audio and text chat, bulletin boards, list servers, massively multiplayer online games, virtual worlds, and Weblogs are some of the many technological platforms that young people are using today to communicate with each other. They all offer different approaches to synchronicity, persistence, anonymity, group dynamics, transience, impression formation, deception multimodality, and governing codes of conduct or netiquette. It goes beyond the scope of this chapter to explore each of these different forms of online communication. A young field of study called computer-mediated communication takes this on (Herring, 2002).

Constructs such as Internet social capital (Williams, 2006b) have been developed to understand new technologies as tools to bridge relationships and bond with others. Researchers such as Robert Kraut at Carnegie Mellon University and colleagues (e.g., Kraut et al., 2002) found that contrary to common criticism of Internet communication (e.g., Putnam, 2000), online bonding or online in-group activities do not predict insularity. Furthermore, research found a strong and significant positive relationship between bonding with similar in-group online peers (such as peers who play video games together or share interests and hobbies), bridging to make contact with others unlike oneself, and meeting new people.

Technologies that effectively provide ways for children to communicate not only facilitate social interaction but also promote language and literacy development. This is an essential developmental task for younger children. For example, studies have shown that when playing together at the computer, children speak twice as many words per minute than during other non-technology-related play activities such as play dough and building blocks (New & Cochran, 2007). Research also found that children spend nine times as much time talking to peers while working with computers as they do working on puzzles (Muller & Perlmutter, 1985).

The possibility of extending young children's communicative potential through virtual worlds and multiplayer games also brings the need to focus on safety. Virtual worlds explicitly designed for young children such as Panwapa and Club Penguin are aware of this and only allow children to communicate with others through already made conversational scripts (Beals & Bers, 2009). Disney's massively multiplayer online role-playing game Toontown Online initially restricted its chat feature to a list of predetermined acceptable phrases but then allowed parents the control over the accounts of children under the age of 18. For example, parents can choose either Chat; SpeedChat, which restricts the user to a limited number of preapproved phrases; or SpeedChat Plus, which allows slightly more freedom of expression by restricting the user to a preapproved dictionary of acceptable words.

While this makes sense to prevent potential problems, it also deprives children of the opportunity to learn how to communicate, how to take care of themselves, and how to identify which social connections are desirable and which ones should be avoided. Think of the playground and the playpen metaphors that I discussed in the first part of this book. In the playground children can communicate with many other children and adults, but the risk is higher than in the playpen in our living room. However, although children roam free in the playground, they are not alone. Adults are sitting on benches or watching behind the fences; they are monitoring the kinds of communications their children engage in. At the sign of risk, such as an unknown adult who doesn't seem to belong to the playground scene, attentive parents can jump in. And they do. And they take advantage of that experience to educate the child on how to behave next time something like this happens. Of course, in the virtual world it is not so easy to identify potential risks, especially when young children are left alone in the technological landscape. Thus, many parents seem to welcome a playpen approach to communication: safety above all. Others would rather spend the time talking with young people, listening to their ideas about how the Internet can play a role in promoting connections and its dangers and safe practices.

As children grow, they get out of the playpen, with or without parents' permission. They encounter a large world. They go to bigger schools, they walk on the street on their own, they participate in overnight summer camps, they go to parties where not every child is known to them, and so on. The possibilities of communication grow exponentially. The same happens in the technological landscape. Adolescents use online communication tools, such as instant messaging and social networking sites, "to reinforce existing relationships, both friendships and romantic relationships, and to check out the potential of new entrants into their offline world" (Subrahmanyam & Greenfield, 2008, p. 120). It is the developmental task of a healthy growing child to find ways to connect with others. And she will use any medium at hand to satisfy this need. It is not surprising that popular social media applications, such as Facebook, were started by young people who had the urge to find new ways to connect with others.

However, increased means of communication do not necessarily equate with increased quality of connection. For example, cyberbullying, or the use of a digital medium to send or post text or images intended to hurt or embarrass another person, has received lots of attention in the news. Privacy issues surrounding the monitoring and recording of communication have also become important considerations, especially with teens who are trying to seek autonomy.

Richard Lerner's (2007) work shows that adults can encourage positive connections by having respectful conversations, considering timing and personal space, engaging in shared activities (e.g., communicating through actions), supporting children's efforts to connect to people outside the family, respecting teens' privacy, and creating and following family rituals. The PTD framework encourages adults to explore the multiple ways in which our technological landscape can promote positive connections to others—family members, teachers, friends, coaches, mentors, and people in the community.

Depending on the kind of desired connection, certain technologies might be better than others. For example, e-mail, Skype, and the dozens of photo-sharing programs allow young people to communicate with those who are far away and can be used to strengthen already existing connections. Some families have the ritual of posting online photo albums and sharing them with family members, as a way to welcome each

New Year. Other families create active mailing lists to communicate with distant relatives and share important events, such as birthdays and celebrations, accomplishments, memories about those who have died in the family, and civic activities.

Certain things, such as the location of computers in a public space in the home, might have an impact. Much has been written about Internet safety and how to protect children from the risks of engaging in communicative exchanges that might lead to negative outcomes. Some interventions are funded and initiated by the U.S. government; others, by private industry; and still others, by motivated individuals. For example, researchers such as Sonia Livingstone (2009) and Web sites such as Digital Mom (http://www.digitalmomblog.com/) explore the complex dynamic between online opportunities and online risks. The Facebook Safety Center provides tips for keeping children safe online, and organizations such as StopCyberbullying.org are dedicated to Internet safety, security, and privacy. The National Center for Missing and Exploited Children and its affiliated site, NetSmartz.org, provide information appealing to children and adults using the motto "Educate. Engage. Empower."

A digital landscape that offers the possibility of communicating to form social connections with peers and adults has the potential to promote positive development. As psychologists Subrahmanyam and Greenfield (2008) write: "For today's youth, media technologies are an important social variable and ... physical and virtual worlds are psychologically connected; consequently, the virtual world serves as a playing ground for developmental issues from the physical world" (p. 124). As children grow and develop, their use of the Internet to communicate might follow more or less the same developmental trajectory as what happens offline. They will encounter positive and negative experiences. However, as designers of the digital landscape we will choose technologies that enable children to communicate with others in order to make positive connections. It is worth the risk, just like on the playground.

Vignette 1
"WII" CAN PLAY STAR WARS

By Alyssa Ettinger

David, seven years old, Huntington Beach, Calif.
David is a first grader who loves battling with action figures, playing with his sci-fi BIONICLE LEGOs, and watching the latest Batman episodes on Cartoon Network. On his calmer days, he enjoys a good game of chess,

cooking, and gardening. At school in Huntington Beach, David has been excelling in math, and just this year he began studying fractions and multiplication with an advanced math tutor. On the other hand, David lags behind his classmates in reading comprehension and several aspects of social development. He is a bright, energetic young boy, but he has trouble relating to others and cannot yet fully understand the motivations and consequences behind behaviors. Nonetheless, David has forged several new friendships with boys in his class through a shared love of action hero cartoons. These shows have truly become transmedia content—not only do the boys watch the cartoons together, they also reenact the fighting scenes with action figures in the play room and then virtually take on the heroes' roles in video games.

On his seventh birthday, David was thrilled to receive LEGO Star Wars: The Complete Saga, made for the Wii. As this was one of his first Wii games, he was amazed by the ability of the remote to transfer his arm movements to the swinging of his avatar's light saber. After a few weeks of exploring "Story Mode," in which the player is guided through a series of specific quests that follow the plot progression in the movies, David was able to master the basic aspects of the game. His favorite mode is now "Free Play Mode," in which the player can explore and choose his own quests, managing a team of characters whose unique abilities are each useful in different situations. The two-player function has made the game an instant hit among David's friends during their after-school play dates. In contrast to many of the action video games they are used to, LEGO Star Wars orients the players as teammates rather than opponents. As the self-appointed game "expert," David frequently leads the expeditions, explaining to his friends how to battle through the obstacles alongside his avatar. When an enemy approaches, David and his teammate hurriedly strategize to effectively split up the roles of defense and offense. As they gain experience and skill, they are now beginning to explore new features of the levels and characters, searching for interesting new ways to complete both novel and familiar quests.

Instead of the usual winner and loser following an antagonistic "battle," this game has fostered a new spirit of teamwork between David and his friends—and appears to be providing a gateway to further personal and social development. The game promotes communication between the players in the two-player feature. The players must build upon and respond to each other's voiced ideas off-screen and transfer this shared understanding to coordinate their avatars' movements on-screen. In addition, once players have developed a multidimensional understanding—leading to further competence and confidence in their gaming abilities—the "Free Play Mode" allows players to creatively explore different game levels and design new combinations of characters and strategies to complete quests.

Vignette 2
DEVIANT ART

By Brandon Lee

Vincent, 20 years old, Santa Cruz, Calif.

Meet Vincent. You can tell by his size that he is in high school, and you can tell by his style and demeanor that he is one of those artsy types. He has on thick plastic glasses and just enough stubble to be able to look at a painting in a museum and justify rubbing his chin while wallowing in deep contemplation. His pants hang low, seemingly struggling to avoid revealing the dangers that lie underneath, and it is unclear whether or not his T-shirt, which pays tribute to a cartoon that was canceled in the 1990s, is 15 years old or brand new. Yes, he is definitely one of THOSE artsy types. Vince is a lover of art and all things art, and he one day aspires to be an animator for Pixar. Now, he spends his time drawing cartoons for the school newspaper, teaching art classes, or sketching things on his own free time.

He knows he is a good artist, but everyone else knows he's a great artist. His simple, cute, and overly cartoony representation of the world around him makes everyone feel happy. His re-creations of popular video game characters, drawn from a new perspective, make gamers and nerds everywhere giggle. However, Vince is focused on how he just cannot draw girls correctly or how his style will never be viewed favorably from an artistic perspective. Eight years later, and a degree in computer science with a concentration in animation from the University of Southern California in hand, many internships, and a job as a technical director at Nickelodeon later, Vince is still wearing that same shirt with a *ThunderCats* cartoon logo on it. His glasses are now held together by glue, and his pants have risen slightly. He still does not work for Pixar but instead works for Lucasfilm on the *Star Wars: The Clone Wars* TV series, where the scenes he has animated will begin to surface in 2011. His drawings, now much more refined, adhere to the same style and silliness of his older work. After eight years, he never abandoned his art style or his desire to become an animator, when many often give up their ambitions to chase art as a career.

Although Vince always had a strong will and desire to become an animator and most likely would not have been stopped by anything, there were factors that helped him along the way. One of those factors could be found in the online community of deviantART. Imagine a social networking site like Myspace, where every user has a shared interest as pervasive as art, which transcends into many media and meanings for many different people, about 11 million in fact. What separates deviantART from other social networking sites is the ability to post one's personal artwork on the site. This online community is as diverse as the world it represents, with people who like to draw, take photographs, create 3-D models, make flash animations, or sculpt. Furthermore, there are as many different styles as there are users, as each artist takes on his or her own perspective on art.

Users not only post artwork on their pages for people to see but also allow others to comment on their work. On this Web site, praise is appreciated, but constructive criticism is encouraged. Users "friend" or follow people if they share or like similar art styles. Exploring Vince's deviantART profile, you can track his development. His pictures back in high school linger in the archives, with one having to go back many pages to find them. Here one will find redone pictures of cartoons or game characters and Christmas Cards for his ex-girlfriend. Comments abound, such as one by the user pdRydia:

> I'd like to say something deep and meaningful, useful or some such ... but, you know. The usual excuses. You've really captured the feel of the game, too, with the colors and comic style. I really appreciate the simple expressions, which are still so unique—Poo's face cracks me up something awful. And, of course, Mr. Saturn.

A comment by another user, JimTscout, is much simpler and much more concise but elicits the same message—"Nice."

As one progresses, Vince's 3-D work starts to become more commonplace. It starts with simple 3-D models. As he had just started with his animation work in college, users offer advice such as "try cell-shading it instead," suggested by user VezCom. Quickly, the works are no longer just 3-D models but screen shots from animations Vince has created. And as his work progresses, the community he has found in deviantART continues to support and scaffold him whenever he needs it, providing insight whenever they can.

DeviantART has created an environment comprised of people who share a similar interest; they provide feedback to each other, learn from each other, and teach each other so that everyone can build upon their own work. Before the Internet, it would have been much more difficult finding a group of people who share similar interests. Perhaps if Vince went to an art school, he would have had an artistic community to work and grow within, but artists don't just go to art school. The power of an online community like deviantART is that it brings in different people from all over the world without one having to move away from the comfort of one's desk. Finally, someone in Oslo can give praise to the work of a 20-year-old aspiring animator in California.

Vignette 3
VIRTUAL SUPPORT FOR SIBLINGS

By Kathryn A. Cantrell

Maria, 16 years old, Galveston, Tex.

Maria, a vivacious teenage girl, lives in Galveston with her parents and her younger sister, Vivian, who is experiencing childhood cancer. Maria loves to go shopping and plays on her high school volleyball team. During the week, though, you often find her absent from school, caring for her younger sister while her parents both work two jobs to afford the medical care. Vivian, six, is energetic and positive, despite her leukemia diagnosis. Maria escorts Vivian through doctor's appointments and medical procedures, being a consistent and caring role model for her sister.

One summer, Maria and Vivian both attended Camp for All, a camp for children with cancer, blood disorders, and their siblings. It was their first year to attend camp, and the two were placed in separate cabins, a stressful event for Vivian, who was showing signs of homesickness. Maria, throughout the week, would visit Vivian's cabin, checking in on her younger sister and making sure she was having fun. The camp environment became a niche for Maria during the week. She quickly became a cabin leader and was seen initiating cabin cheers and leading the other girls through activities. She made many friends at camp and was open with others about her experience as a sibling and what it's like to navigate the health care system for Vivian.

At the end of the week, all the youth were introduced to a virtual community for Camp for All campers. The online virtual world was called Zora Camp4All and allowed campers to keep in touch during the remainder of the year. Password protected and monitored, the site offered a safe resource for campers to continue sharing stories and offering support through medical illness. The virtual community also provided a psychosocial curriculum aimed at addressing hopefulness, a construct used within the Camp for All culture.

Maria eagerly participated in Zora Camp4All and was online for multiple hours a day. During one of the group's first sessions, Maria spoke about being a sibling of a child with cancer. She said, "There is support for my parents at the hospital because they go to a support group and there is support for Vivian because she has playrooms and doctors caring for her. But there's nothing for me." During the weeks of virtual camp, Maria religiously attended the sessions and openly talked about her experience with cancer. However, it was during one of the final virtual group sessions that Maria opened up about more than just illness. During the online sessions, participants were asked to design an object within the Zora virtual world that represented what hope meant to them. Many of the youth constructed objects that alluded to hospital stays and chemotherapy. Maria, however, focused on something else. Using an image of the sun, Maria constructed an object to represent hopefulness. Within the object's description, it read: "Hope is the sunshine after a hurricane."

When she shared the object with the group, Maria spoke about her family's move from New Orleans to Galveston after Hurricane Katrina. She explained how difficult it was for her to leave her friends at home and be a new student at a large high school. She also spoke about how stressful it was to both move and care for Vivian. It was a strong testament to the multiple life stressors experienced by many teenagers today. At the end of the virtual session, though, she concluded with: "I am happier here. I've made better friends in Texas than I had in New Orleans. And my sister is healthier. At first, I was devastated but now I love it even more." Maria, eloquent and mature, hopes to one day become a social worker to help other children like Vivian while they are in the hospital. By pointing out the brighter side to life's challenges, Maria will continue being a source of optimism and hope for her younger sister.

CHAPTER 8

Collaboration to Form Caring Networks

Following on the previous chapter, this section focuses on the different ways in which the digital landscape can promote collaborative endeavors. Although there is a great amount of research looking at how computer-supported collaboration has an impact on productivity and learning, this chapter focuses on collaboration as a way to promote caring, defined in this context as the willingness to respond to the needs of other individuals, to assist others, and to use technology as means to help others. This chapter suggests that tools for collaboration are essential for enabling the formation of caring networks.

Collaboration is a process where two or more people or organizations work together to realize shared goals. The low cost and nearly instantaneous sharing of ideas, knowledge, and skills facilitated by the Internet have made collaborative processes dramatically easier. The nonhierarchical structure of the technology also allows for new forms of self-organization and leadership to emerge through these collaborations. Collaboration can happen across the ocean or with the neighbor next door, with people we already know or with those who share a niche interest and meet online with the sole purpose of working together. In technical terms, collaboration can be colocated or geographically distributed, and individuals can collaborate synchronously (at the same time) or asynchronously (not at the same time).

Our digital landscape is populated by a broad range of tools that enable people to work together in all of these different ways: social networking, instant messaging, team spaces, Web sharing, blogs, wikis, and audio and video conferencing. Many of today's popular software is produced in a collaborative manner by large numbers of people working mostly without traditional hierarchical organization or financial compensation. For example, products resulting from these collaborations include the Linux operating system; Slashdot, a news and announcements Web site; and Wikipedia, an online collaborative encyclopedia.

Most specifically, the field of computer-supported cooperative work (CSCW) focuses on how technology can support and coordinate people in their work (Grudin, 1994). CSCW is a design-oriented academic field that brings together social psychologists, sociologists, anthropologists, and computer scientists, among others, to identify needed design features to support such cooperative work and evaluate outcomes. For example, researchers have focused on levels of awareness, appropriation, organizational memory, visualization techniques, and more.

Most recently, those working on the design and study of educational technologies created a scholarly community concerned with computer-supported collaborative learning (CSCL). This is a pedagogical approach that looks at how learning can be best enhanced by providing mechanisms to support learners to engage in a common task where each individual depends on and is accountable to each other. This approach shifts the process of cognition as residing within the head of one individual to the view that cognition is situated within a particular community of learning or practice (Lave & Wenger, 1991). This is heavily rooted in Vygotsky's (1978) inherent social nature of learning. Technologies inspired by the CSCL paradigm must take seriously the need to provide tools for communities to engage in all three C's that deal with the interpersonal domain: communication, collaboration, and community building. For example, new programming environments, such as Scratch, have vibrant online communities of sharing, contribution, and collaboration (Resnick et al., 2009).

Research shows that when children are using computers, they are more likely to ask other children for advice and help, even if an adult is present, thus increasing collaboration toward positive socialization (Wartella & Jennings, 2000), and they are also more likely to engage in new forms of collaboration (New & Cochran, 2007). For example, in the TangibleK robotics program run by my DevTech research group at Tufts University, we have developed a low-tech pedagogical tool, called "collaboration web," to help children become aware of their collaborative patterns (Bers, 2010b). At the beginning of each day of work, along with their design journals and their robotic kits, children are given a personalized printout with their photograph in the center of the page and the photographs and names of all other children in the class arranged in a circle surrounding their own photo. Throughout the day, when the teacher prompts students to do so, each child uses the collaboration web and draws a line from his or her own photo to the photo of the children he or she had collaborated with. For this purpose, collaboration is defined as getting or giving help with their project, programming together, lending or borrowing materials, or working together on a common task. At the end of the week, children write or draw "thank-you cards" to the children whom they have collaborated with the most.

For young children who are in a developmental process of learning how to work with others, it is important to design a digital landscape that includes both technical supports and social supports to encourage collaboration. This is essential to promote social and pro-social development. However, not all collaborative interactions around the technology lead to the formation of caring relationships and caring individuals. Richard Lerner, in his book *The Good Teen*, remembers his grandmother's way to define the concept of caring. He recalls showing her his report card and her response: "This is very nice. Getting good grades is important. But what is really important is being a mensch!" (2007, p. 165). This Yiddish word refers to a good person, someone who thinks not only of himself but of others, someone who cares about issues and people outside his direct small world, someone who listens, someone with a "big heart," someone who has compassion. According to the PTD framework, the ultimate goal of participating in collaborative endeavors in our technological landscape is to become a mensch. In the process, we might increase productivity and learning opportunities, but from a positive developmental perspective, the goal of collaboration is to form caring relationships.

Vignette 1

FIGHTING TO WIN: BUILDING CONNECTION THROUGH LIVEJOURNAL

By Jeewon Kim

Laura, 16 years old, Akron, Ohio

Laura is a 16-year-old high school sophomore who resides in Akron, Ohio, a suburb of Cleveland. Her father is an electrical engineer, and her mother stays at home to look after Laura's baby sister, Grace. Laura's older sister, Cynthia, attends a university near Chicago, Illinois. Her parents hope for her to finish high school and follow Cynthia's example. Gymnastics were Laura's passion as a child. Placed on the balance beam as a toddler, she trained extensively through her early childhood and elementary years. She competed at the regional level and once even advanced with her team to the state tournament.

Now an adolescent, Laura no longer competes and is more or less without an extracurricular pursuit in her life.

Laura was forced to quit gymnastics in middle school as a consequence of her struggle with anorexia. An estimated 1%–5% of adolescent women in the United States suffer from this disorder in which individuals refrain from eating in an attempt to lose weight and satisfy their distorted body image. Legitimate cases of anorexia nervosa are classified by the *DSM-IV* as ones in which individuals fall below 85% of their expected body weight. At 13 years old, Laura met this criterion and endured a brief hospitalization to confront her disorder. Today, at 16, Laura maintains an average body weight, but the struggle is not over. She's unable to return to the world of gymnastics, both for lack of practice and because of the risk of exposure to the competitive, weight-obsessed world that drove her to starve herself in the first place. Laura sees her school therapist from time to time when her anxieties are triggered. More regularly though, she finds solace in a digital medium—her LiveJournal.

LiveJournal is an online journal service (oftentimes referred to as a "blog") with a self-described "emphasis on user interaction." The service is free, although paying members receive access to premium features (e.g., extensive journal-"style" customization). Individual members can record both public and private content in their personal journals. LiveJournal users can meet other users by joining "communities," or *group* journals in which multiple users can post entries of public or private nature (in this case, "private" indicates that the content is for the group's eyes only). "Communities" must have at least one or more "maintainers" who serve in a supervising and administrative role.

Laura is a member of a community called "proanorexia: World's Largest Pro Anorexia Site 24 Hr Posting." The title of the group is purposely misleading. *Pro Anorexia* (or *Pro Ana*) refers to individuals who encourage each other's disorders by posting pictures of "thinspiration" and organizing "group fasts." This particular LiveJournal community of 16,489 members uses its title to draw in men and women who are anorexic and looking for like-minded individuals and then surprises them with a site full of positive support and strategies to fight the disorder. The maintainer, "fighting2win," includes a list of rules at the entrance to the community, first and foremost of which is written in bold typeface and reads: "***ALWAYS MAKE OTHER MEMBERS FEEL WELCOME.***" The group intends to serve as a connective network for those suffering with or recovering from anorexia, as well as those who have won their struggles and are looking to counsel others. The group maintains strict guidelines outlawing the posting of "triggers" and the "teaching of damaging behavior." Users who violate these terms are banned from the community without question.

Laura's participation in this group has had a considerable impact on her recovery from anorexia. She logs in to the community for an hour or so each day after school, and now three years after her hospitalization, she has begun to provide counseling and support to other teens who are still entrenched in the disorder. Laura feels a great sense of pride at now being able to serve and support others in a network that once served her and helped save her life. The collaborative nature of "proanorexia" is an excellent means toward connection between individuals. Users from all over the United States and beyond are able to unite in the face of their common obstacles. LiveJournal truly fulfills the promise of its name and promotes healthy living.

Vignette 2
IS HE OKAY? ASK FACEBOOK

By Jeewon Kim

Peter, 17 years old, Alexandria, Va.
Peter is a 17-year-old high school student who attends the prestigious Thomas Jefferson High School for Science and Technology in Alexandria, Virginia, minutes outside of the nation's capital. Peter is a senior, and like his classmates, he has lofty hopes for college and fills his day with Advanced Placement classes and extracurricular activities that guide him toward that next major milestone in his life. The Shakespeare Troupe is Peter's greatest passion. He participates as both actor and student director and feels fortunate to have fallen in love with the Bard at such an early age. Rehearsals for shows—this year, *Twelfth Night* and *The Merchant of Venice*—dominate Peter's after-school hours.

At home, Peter's family sits down together to dinner each night and sometimes catches a favorite TV show or two before Peter commits his evening to his homework. In between BC Calculus problem sets and Spanish flash cards, Peter updates his Facebook profile to pass the time. Peter adds "friends," posts messages on "walls," and updates his "status" to advertise upcoming play performances.

On April 16, 2007, tragedy struck the nearby Virginia Polytechnic Institute and State University (a.k.a. Virginia Tech). A young gunman took the lives of 32 victims and wounded many others before taking his own life. More than 15% of graduating seniors from Peter's high school attend Virginia Tech. Upon hearing of the breaking news, panic struck Peter's heart as he remembered Darren, his costar from last year's *Love's Labour's Lost*, now a freshman at Virginia Tech. Calls to Darren's cell phone were fruitless—much like in New York City on 9/11, the cell phone towers in Blacksburg, Virginia, were jammed with calls from anxious friends and family desperate to hear from their loved ones. Peter then turned to a seemingly unlikely solution—his Facebook.

Darren's Facebook profile displayed the following "status update" posted 30 minutes before: "I'm okay. Pray for us." Displayed on Darren's "wall" were messages of support and prayer from his Facebook "friends." Peter then checked the profiles of several other friends at Virginia Tech and found similar postings.

Despite the ongoing tragedy, Peter breathed a little bit easier knowing that his loved ones, at least, were safe and secure in their dorm rooms.

Facebook continued to provide a medium for networks of caring and support in the weeks that followed the tragedy. Dozens of "groups" honoring the deceased were created, garnering thousands of members each. Tens of thousands of status updates from students across the country declared, "We are all Hokies," the Virginia Tech mascot. Thousands upon thousands more students updated their profile photos to display the Virginia Tech emblem intertwined with that of their own institution as a show of solidarity with the victims and their loved ones.

In the wake of tragedy, Peter's story and Facebook demonstrated the enormous potential of the digital medium to facilitate collaboration toward the formation of caring networks. Students utilized a digital social-networking tool to create a united front in support of their peers in Blacksburg. Many parents created Facebook pages in the aftermath, citing that their children's friends were able to confirm their safety before they were because of the Web site. Virginia Tech students were truly touched by the outpouring of digital support sent their way—the Internet (and Facebook, in particular) let them know that not only their friends and family but also their entire country was watching out for them.

Vignette 3
BUILDING ROBOTS, MAKING FRIENDS

By Jared Matas

Judah, six years old, Boston, Mass.
Judah is a six-year-old kindergartner at Boston's Jewish Community Day School (JCDS). His parents report that at home, he spends hours playing independently, in particular putting together complex LEGO kits designed for much older children. Judah has difficulty negotiating social interactions with his peers, and recess is often a source of great frustration for him. His parents chose to enroll Judah in JCDS because of its reputation for attention to individual learning needs, as well as the emphasis on *menshlechkit* (being a good person). Judah's parents want to continue to encourage his academic learning, but they are beginning to be concerned with the frequency that Judah gets into conflicts with his classmates.

This fall, Judah's class participated in a LEGO robotic engineering unit, using the TangibleK curriculum and materials. The students learned to program their LEGO robots using CHERP, a tangible–graphical hybrid programming language designed specifically for young children. Children using CHERP physically construct programs by connecting interlocking wooden blocks with bright colored labels that both a computer and a young child can recognize. Once the student has built a program by connecting a series of wooden blocks, he or she loads the program onto a robot via a laptop computer. A Webcam attached to the computer takes a picture of the blocks and then transmits it to a robot using a tower plugged into the laptop's USB port. The students quickly learn the steps and become proficient at building programs and loading the programs on their robots.

Judah was looking forward to "doing LEGO robots at school." He had a lot of experience with his LEGO kits at home and was curious to see what he could build with LEGO robots. He was expecting to excel at this material, as he considers himself a "LEGO expert." The first lesson, however, was very stressful. After the teacher handed each pair of students a plastic box that contained the LEGO parts, Judah grabbed the box out of his partner's hands, ripped off the lid, and then declared in disappointment, "I can't do this, there are no instructions!"

"How am I going to build the wheels to my car if I don't have that axel?" Judah said, as he grabbed the part out of his partner's hand.

As the two boys tussled over the piece, their box turned over, sending all the pieces to the ground in a noisy crash.

"See what you made me do!" Judah told his partner, as he grabbed a handful of pieces and stormed off to a different corner of the classroom.

After a few minutes, the teacher approached Judah, who was already engrossed in his LEGO construction. After praising Judah for his building, the teacher discussed the interaction with his partner. "You are already an expert builder," the teacher said. "What I want you to work on for next time is sharing the materials with your classmates."

At the end of each lesson there is a "Technology Circle." This is an opportunity for the students to share their work and for the teacher to review key concepts. The teacher uses this sharing to emphasize not just computer programming concepts specific to this unit but also elements of the social curriculum that pervade all aspects of the kindergarten program throughout the year. After Judah showed his LEGO vehicle to the class, the teacher asked him if he was willing to be a helper for other students who were having a hard time getting the wheels to stay attached to the robot. Judah nodded his head. "Now we know that if anyone needs help with Sturdy Building, Judah is a good person to ask for help." The teacher created an opportunity for a positive social interaction for Judah, using Judah's expertise with LEGO building.

The next student to share had only a few pieces of LEGO, loosely connected. She wanted to pass on her turn, but the teacher insisted, "I noticed that Sarah and her partner worked really well today. Could you tell us about that, Sarah?" The teacher deliberately highlighted a pair that cooperated more successfully than Judah and his pair, immediately after Judah's turn, so that Judah could learn from that experience. Sarah had a harder time talking about it—she was embarrassed by the contrast between her simple robot and the construction that Judah showed the class. The teacher provided some reminders: "When you first sat down with your partner, you both wanted to build on that red square platform. What did you do next?" Sarah told the class how she and her partner peacefully divided the LEGO pieces in their box. The teacher celebrated this interaction, with even more praise than Judah received for his LEGO building.

Judah will still need reminders in the next lesson about sharing the materials, but he has received a strong message about the value of cooperation. The teacher celebrated both a successful final product and successful teamwork. Positive models were shared, with encouragement to follow that example next time. The LEGO robotics curriculum is taught in lessons that only occur twice a week. The social curriculum, however, is present throughout the day, every day.

The following day at recess, Judah and another student raced for a soccer ball. His teacher saw this and could build on the language from the Technology Circle to encourage Judah to make a good choice. A student will need multiple experiences before fully internalizing the value of collaboration and being able to consistently display positive behavior choices. Emphasizing proper conduct during technology lessons creates one more opportunity to encourage the development of this habit of mind.

CHAPTER 9

Community Building as Contribution

Hillel, one of the greatest sages and scholars in the Jewish tradition, who lived in Jerusalem during the time of King Herod and the Roman emperor Augustus, is attributed with the wise saying: "If I am not for myself, then who will be for me? And if I am only for myself, then what am I? And if not now, when?" (Ethics of the Fathers 1:14). This old proverb summarizes the concept of community building. Both individual and society need to flourish together.

As we have seen in the previous two chapters on the C's of communication and collaboration, a digital landscape that promotes positive youth development should support the human need for establishing and sustaining social relationships. The C of contribution takes this a step further. It reminds us that new technologies can and must provide mechanisms for giving back to others, to contribute to make our world a better place. Richard Lerner's work shows that when young people are competent and confident, when they have a strong sense of character and they can connect with and care about others, they will also be able to contribute to society. All six C's are interrelated, but according to Lerner, the C of contribution makes them all come together and is "the glue that creates healthy human development" (2007, p. 183). While contribution is an internal asset, a natural capacity of all human beings, new technologies can facilitate behaviors such as community building that lead to contribution in the form of community service, activism, and advocacy.

Scholars have different terms to talk about community building and contribution. For example, they use the umbrella concept of civic engagement. Some conceive civic engagement as simply being a good neighbor, obeying rules, and participating in the community, while others think of it as engagement with political processes, such as voting

(Sherrod, Flanagan, & Youniss, 2002). The concept of civic engagement goes beyond the procedural aspects of democracy to a model that embraces the many facets of a deliberative and participatory democracy. Civic engagement can take many forms, from individual voluntarism to organizational involvement to electoral participation (Keeter, Zukin, Andolina, & Jenkins, 2002; Montgomery, 2008). It can include efforts to directly address an issue or work with others in a community to solve a problem or interact with the institutions of representative democracy. We don't need to be of voting age to engage in civic activities. Civic engagement encompasses a range of activities, such as working in a soup kitchen, serving on a neighborhood association, writing a letter to an elected official, organizing a protest, fund-raising for a cause, and so forth. A civically engaged individual has the ability, agency, and opportunity to make a change in his community. The range of communities, the scope of the change, and the possibilities for making it happen vary according to the age of the individual, among many other factors.

Our digital landscape offers many opportunities for civic engagement. Researchers contend that the Internet can be a venue for helping young people develop a sense of voluntarism and activism, for engaging in new forms of civic activities such as online petitioning and civic dialogues, and for promoting traditional types of civic activities such as voting (Bers, 2008c, 2008e; Blumler & Coleman, 2001; Cassell, 2002; Cassell, Huffaker, Tversky, & Ferriman, 2006; Earl & Schussman, 2008; Montgomery, 2008; Montgomery, Gottlieb-Robles, & Larson, 2004; Rheingold, 2008). While several efforts try to understand the potential of youth as e-citizens, the challenge remains in how to promote participation not only in the virtual world but also in the face-to-face world. Some work is starting to tap into this challenge. For example, TakingITGlobal is a popular online community that engages youth in connecting with others to take action in their local and global communities. TakingITGlobal, like other similar virtual communities, puts effort into using virtual worlds to make a difference in the face-to-face world (Raynes-Goldie & Walker, 2008).

The Internet provides a new way for youth to create communities that extend beyond geographic boundaries, to engage in civic and volunteering activities across local communities and national frontiers, to learn about political life, and to experience the challenges of democratic participation. Video games also tap into this potential by providing opportunities for young people to contribute to "participatory cultures" with low barriers to expression and civic engagement (Jenkins, 2009). For example, in 2004 a network of nonprofit directors, game developers, artists, and academics committed to social change through gaming came together to form the Games for Change (G4C) movement, a branch of serious games focused on social issues and social change. Since then, G4C organizes a yearly event dedicated to showcasing video games for social change—games about poverty, global conflict, and climate change—and bringing together "socially responsible game makers."

This growing work on "serious" games (Bers, 2010c; Gee, 2003; Kahne et al., 2008; Squire, 2011) found that several aspects of video games play parallel the kinds of civic learning opportunities found to promote civic engagement in other settings. For example, video games that engage youth in simulations of civic and political action, consideration of controversial issues, and participation in groups of shared interests, all activities that are done in school settings as part of civics education programs, are effective in encouraging civic participation (Kahne et al., 2008). While some games have content that is directly relevant to civics, such as SimCity and Civilization, which engage players in simulations of civic processes, other video games lack explicit relevant civic content but still might promote habits of mind that are critical for civic life (Bers, 2010c). For example, multiplayer games in the virtual world such as World of Warcraft and EverQuest engage players in governance, team building, leadership, and organizational processes.

A recent survey conducted by the Pew Internet and American Life Project found that more than four in 10 youths say that video games have taught them about a societal problem (Lenhart et al., 2008) and that game-playing youth were more likely to search for information about current events online, advocate for political candidates, and raise money for charity. Furthermore, Kahne, Middaugh, and Evans (2008) have found that "the stereotype of the antisocial game" is not reflected in the data from their study, as "youth who play games frequently are just as civically and politically active as those who play games infrequently" (p. 27). These researchers examined civic gaming experiences in relation to civics outcomes and found that the quantity of game play is not strongly related to civic and political engagement but that some aspects of the social context of game play are related to civic outcomes, specifically playing games with others. This is not surprising; social relationships are at the core of the C's of contribution and community building.

Virtual worlds can be purposefully designed to provide civic education for young people. For example, Quest Atlantis, developed by Sasha Barab and colleagues at Indiana University, embeds civic learning opportunities in the quest for children, ages nine–16, to find solutions to the problems faced by a fictional world called Atlantis. The virtual world is explicitly designed to enhance the lives of children while helping them grow into knowledgeable, responsible, and empathetic adults (Barab et al., 2005). With my own work, the Zora virtual world provides a safe "social laboratory" for youth to experiment with some of the skills and attitudes needed to become good citizens (Bers, 2008c; Bers & Chau, 2006, 2010).

For example, we have used Zora in a pre-orientation program at Tufts University called Active Citizenship Through Technology to encourage incoming first-year students to explore the civic responsibility of a college campus and the relationship to its neighbors (Bers, 2008c; Bers & Chau, 2010). In this three-day pilot program, which was run in two consecutive years, incoming first-year students used Zora to design and inhabit a *Virtual Campus of the Future*. While building the different locations on the campus, they expressed concerns and ideas about community issues of interest to them. For example, they built the "Campus safety center," which offers

> a shuttle service for 18 hours a day followed by a campus cab system that goes anywhere in a 5 mile radius of the campus, and the "Jumbo Appetite," a dining hall where themed meals are served and a suggestion box where requests for particular foods can be made.

They also discussed issues such as student life, policies/rules for graduation, the Internet, administration, and student services. The following is an excerpt of an online conversation in which students discussed funding for students' clubs:

> PETER: Are we going to have fun student clubs? Do clubs have to give back to the community?
> MELANIE: If you are giving back to the community, should you get more money?
> ALAN: Should we fund the clubs?
> PETER: Every year, they give their proposal ... then they decide ... and get their permission.
> DAVID: If you are giving back to the community, you should get money. Why put money into clubs?
> PETER: If it lasts then that is good; but if you are new, you start-off with the minimum amount.

This excerpt shows civic engagement conceived as a process of becoming involved with the civic life of campus, such as assigning internal budgets or developing policies that would be best for students. In a test-driven educational atmosphere in which most schools cannot devote resources and time to increase students' civic participation, the digital landscape has great potential for promoting civic engagement. While participation in virtual life does not replace traditional civic actions, research shows that adults are more likely to vote and be engaged in the civic sphere if, as youths, they were involved in community-based organizations or extracurricular activities (Verba, Schlozman, & Brady, 1995; Youniss, McLellan, & Yates, 1997). As the Internet is becoming a new way for youth to form community-based organizations and to spend a big portion of their after-school time, it is plausible that future research will show that youth who are more active online will also grow into more engaged contributors to society.

Vignette 1
RELAY FOR LIFE: USING THE WEB TO SAVE LIVES

by Jeewon Kim

Phillip, 18 years old, San Luis Obispo, Calif.
Phillip is an 18-year-old high school senior from San Luis Obispo, California, a town on the central California coastline. Phillip will be attending community college in the fall and is thrilled to be wrapping up four successful years of high school. Phillip's girlfriend, Ana, will be attending a university in New England in the fall. Having dated for three years and now unsure of their future, the two are looking to enjoy their last months of childhood together and take their relationship one day at a time.

Phillip plays defensive end for the football team in the fall and is a member of the varsity lacrosse team in the spring. While not a star player, Phillip has enjoyed sports for his whole life and has made many of his best friends on the field. When not wearing his team uniform, Phillip maintains a seemingly unlikely hobby—Web design. Phillip enrolled in a New Media elective in the eighth grade and developed an interest in the Internet that never let up. His final project in that course, a San Diego Chargers fan site, came out quite well and inspired him to continue to explore the world of Web design. A unique turn of events his sophomore year would come to make his newfound hobby a meaningful skill and important contribution.

Five months into Phillip and Ana's relationship, Ana's mother was diagnosed with breast cancer. Ana and her family were rocked by this development, and Ana looked to Phillip for support during this difficult time. That spring, inspired by a loved one's struggle, Phillip was moved to participate in his high school's Relay for Life. Relay for Life (or "Relay," for short) is the principal fund-raising event of the American Cancer Society (ACS). It offers everyone in a community an opportunity to unite in the fight against cancer. The event itself consists of teams of people taking turns walking or running around a track or path for up to 24 hours. These teams have fun at the activity and more important, raise funding and awareness about cancer in the months preceding the Relay itself. Relay for Life particularly honors survivorship of cancer with an emotional candle-lit ceremony in which those fighting and those lost to the battle with cancer are honored. More than 3.5 million Americans participate in the ACS Relay every year, and the event now spans 19 countries outside of U.S. borders.

In the modern age, the Internet is a principal fund-raising tool, and Relay is no different. The ACS provides a Web site template for Relay participants to encourage friends and family to make donations toward their team's fund-raising goal. Pictures of past Relays can be posted, and standard donation e-mails can be sent en masse to address books. Given Phillip's background with Web design, he took his participation in Relay to the next step. Using the Relay model as a reference, he designed his own interactive Web site to raise awareness about both the ACS and his participation in the Relay. Phillip's site included extensive information about living with and fighting cancer, as well as the story of Ana's mother, with her permission. Friends and family were awestruck by a high school student's commitment to the cause, and Phillip raised more funds that year than anyone else on his team.

In the years that followed, Phillip continued to participate with the ACS in a greater capacity, and his Web site evolved along the way. Phillip created a blog for Ana's mother through which she could record her struggle and serve as an inspiration to readers. His senior year, Phillip and Ana served as the coordinators for their high school's Relay for Life. Web design allowed for Phillip to make an outstanding contribution both to his loved ones and to all those individuals fighting cancer. Phillip served as a principal community builder for the ACS in his hometown. Without the Internet, Phillip would not have been able to raise awareness so readily and to move the hearts of friends and family across the nation. Regardless of Phillip and Ana's future as a couple, they will continue to be teammates in their fight for survivorship, however far apart.

Vignette 2
CREATING A WEB SITE, CREATING COMMUNITY

By R. Jordan Crouser

Kit, 23 years old, and Ryan, 20 years old, Boston, Mass.
For the most part, Kit and Ryan are typical 20-something roommates. They're fresh out of undergrad and have recently moved to the Boston area for graduate school and to find work, respectively. They've been friends for the past year and a half, having met through an a cappella group at school. Apart from music and school, Kit and Ryan have one thing in common: they are both

transgender. For them, this means that although they were labeled girls at birth, they feel strongly connected to a more masculine gender presentation. Having settled into their preferred gender roles over the span of a few years and having recently moved to a new city, they are for the most part invisible members of the transgender community.

Relatively introverted in his day-to-day life, Ryan spends a good amount of his free time surfing the Internet. One evening, he reads on a friend's blog that a popular online resource for transgender people looking for health care providers is no longer available. Both Ryan and Kit have used this resource extensively in the past, and so he decides to investigate.

A few more clicks, and he has confirmed this rumor. This particular resource has been increasingly unreliable for the past several years, and it appears that it has finally fallen into such disrepair that its founders have decided to take it permanently offline. Unfortunately, while not well maintained, this site was also the only one of its kind. Because of this, many people in the transgender community are concerned about where they will be able to go to find the information they need on transgender-friendly health care providers.

> "Looks like Transster is down for good."
> "Oh, man. That's too bad. Saw it coming though...."
> Kit goes back to his homework. There is a short silence, and then Ryan asks:
> "Hey . . . how hard is it to build a site like that, do you think?"

They decide to take a crack at creating a new online resource to replace the one that has disappeared, and it doesn't take long before the young men are intently committed to the project. While Ryan registers a new domain name and collects as much of the old site information as he can find, Kit sets to work designing and building his first database-driven Web site. He teaches himself how to make a reliable online registration system and how to prevent unauthorized redistribution of the content people post. They design a logo, add in the content Ryan has collected, and even add an online forum to make it easier for people to ask questions and connect with one another.

Seventeen hours and a generous amount of caffeine later, they unveil their new Web site to the online community. A few friends agree to spread the word, and on the first day the site gets 122 visits, mostly from people in the Boston metro area. Several people post in the forum that they're excited to see where the new site goes, and Kit and Ryan are pleased that their harebrained, late-night project has been well received. Little do they realize that their site will rapidly grow to be one of the most popular online resources for transgender people.

At the time of this writing, their site has over 16,000 members registered from 156 different countries. There are active members on every inhabited continent, and the site has had over 100,000 visits and 500,000 page views since it was launched in 2009. Kit and Ryan have been contacted by health care providers wishing to have their practices listed as transgender-friendly. They have presented at transgender identity conferences, have met several of the world's most prominent transgender speakers, and have connected with other transgender people across the globe. Through this site, these young men empowered their community, facilitated communication across geographic barriers, and raised awareness about some of the unique challenges in health care facing the transgender community.

Vignette 3
ONGOING CONTRIBUTIONS ACROSS THE WORLD

By Hannah Gogel

Allison, 18 years old, Somerville, Mass.
Allison is a first-year college student selected to go on a service trip. She flies with a group of 20 college students, stopping on two continents, and lands in Kigali, Rwanda. The students take an hour-long bus ride on bumpy dirt roads and through small villages to arrive at their destination. Allison spends 10 days at a youth village filled with students ranging from age 14 to 20. Every student there is an orphan of the 1994 genocide. There are 150 students. Every day Allison learns a little more about each of their separate dreams and interests. Some want to be astronauts; others, doctors. They want to hear about Chris Brown and pop culture in the United States. Allison tries to give them all the information they ask for, from political questions to American slang, but 10 days is only enough time to give them a glimpse.

While the Rwandans learn about the United States, Allison and her friends learn about Rwanda—history, songs, dances. Allison goes every night to meet with some of the adults at the village to learn some vocabulary in Kinyarwanda. Allison and her group decide that the students need to be able to stay in touch. There are about 10 computers in the village, and maybe half of the students have e-mail. Each visiting student helps the Rwandans create Facebook accounts. The Internet is slow; Facebook allows the students to load a page of contact information from multiple people, instead of loading one e-mail from one person at a time. After just over a week of tutoring, playing sports, chatting, dancing, and singing with the Rwandan students, Allison's group returns to the United States for summer break.

Throughout the summer and the following year, Allison's group searches for ways to continue their relationship with the students they met from across the world. Articles are written for local newspapers and posted online with videos and photos. Fund-raisers are organized via Facebook groups and access to e-lists of groups with similar interests. With just a few clicks, hundreds of students and community members are informed about the inspiring students in Rwanda. The Internet allows hundreds of people a way to hear about and participate in fund-raisers. A donor is inspired by what a group member posts on the Internet and sponsors an entire science center for the Rwandan students.

Mail outside of the capital of Rwanda isn't very reliable. Facebook becomes the method Allison and her friends use to continue communication with their new friends in Rwanda. They exchange stories and updates on school in both countries. The students share YouTube clips with one another and exchange knowledge of their native languages, varying from Spanish to French to Kinyarwanda. Allison, while chatting with her Rwandan friend on Facebook, teaches him to make a Web site to share his music with the world. Every day, Allison's Facebook news feed has a Rwandan student making a new friendship or sharing a new experience with the worldwide community of Facebook users.

The purpose of Allison's trip, beyond donating shoes and providing tutoring, was to connect students from different places in the world. With the Internet, this service trip's contribution doesn't have to end after 10 days. The students from the United States continue contributing to the youth village, and the youth village continues to contribute to the students and their communities in the United States.

Summary

This second part of the book focused on the behaviors that should be supported by digital landscapes that promote positive youth development. These behaviors, the six C's of content creation, creativity, choice of conduct, communication, collaboration, and community building, become guidelines for designers of the digital landscape. We are all designers, regardless of our expertise and background. We are all invested in making the best for our children. We are not happy with describing what they do with technology; we want to have an impact in making sure that they do the best they can. We intervene. We design.

As designers, we craft environments that encourage children to engage in positive experiences. We complement the affordances of the technologies with practices, curricula, interventions, pedagogies, approaches. Remember: the digital landscape is not a set of tools and technologies but an environment where experiences happen. Let's not confuse the elements of the environment (e.g., virtual worlds, Facebook, Scratch, the Internet, robotics, etc.) with the kinds of experiences that we can have with them. Design is a human-centered activity. However, we need to know what kinds of activities we want to support. Thus, PTD offers the framework of the six C's. The behaviors identified in the framework can happen with and without technology. The challenge is to understand what the affordances of each technology are and what needs to be added.

In the process of engaging in those experiences through creating content, being creative, choosing their conduct, communicating, collaborating, and building community, children also develop internal assets or characteristics that researchers on applied developmental sciences have identified as fundamental for positive development, the six C's of competence, confidence, character, connection, caring, and contribution. Assets have an impact on behaviors and behaviors impact assets in a bidirectional relationship. As designers, we think in terms of design elements, and we ask: What kinds of behaviors should the technological landscape support to promote positive development? How do these behaviors change at different developmental stages? How do these behaviors get translated into technical features that provide mechanisms and processes? Technologies provide ways for us to engage in actions, to do something, to engage in particular behaviors. The six C's of the PTD framework are those behaviors identified as leading to positive outcomes. Although for ease of organization in this book I have chosen to describe each C one at the time, all of them intersect and have an impact on each other (see Figure PII.1). These intersections form the tapestry of a digital landscape that promotes positive development.

Remember the goal of this research endeavor, which I described on the first pages of this book: *"Using technology to help children learn new things to become better people and make a better world."* At the center of this quest is a "why" question, a sense of purpose: becoming better people and making a better world. Thus, the pivotal C's of the PTD framework are choices of conduct to promote character and community building as contribution. I have placed them at both ends. In between, the other C's are at play. All of them are needed as we are looking to design a digital

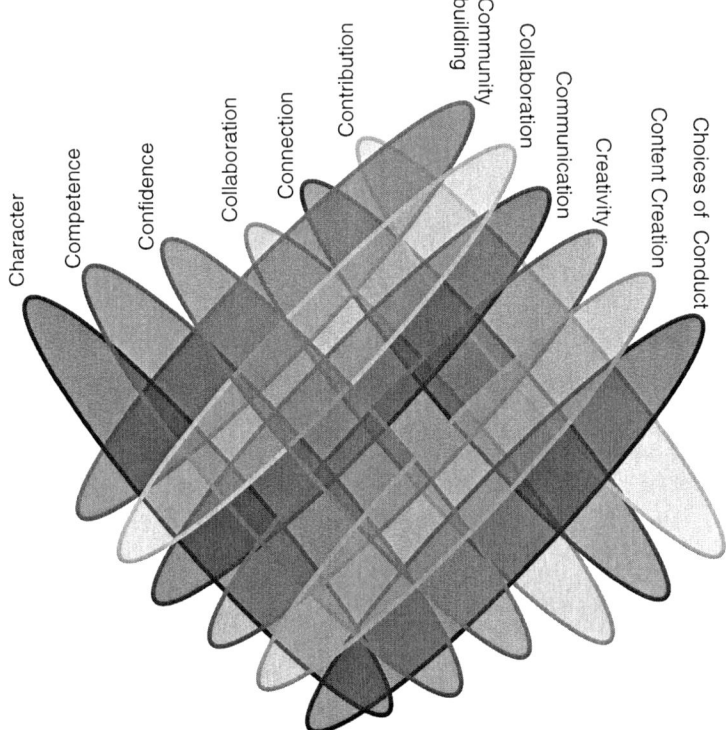

Figure PII.1. The PTD framework as tapestry.

landscape that allows children to create content and develop competence in the technical domain, to express their creativity through digital projects and build confidence in their abilities with new technologies, to communicate with others so that they can build connections with peers and adults that extend beyond face-to-face boundaries, and to collaborate in joint initiatives to show caring and empathy.

PART III

Plotting Learning Trajectories Through Design

OVERVIEW

Some landscapes are natural. Others are purposefully designed to impact their inhabitants. Part I of this book uses different metaphors—the digital playground, the multimedia park, and the palace in time—for understanding the digital world as a space that can promote core developmental milestones from early childhood to high school. Part II of the book goes beyond a descriptive approach. The focus is on how to purposefully design digital landscapes that promote positive youth development. It offers a theoretical framework, PTD, to design digital experiences that engage children in technology-mediated behaviors, the six C's: content creation, creativity, choice of conduct, communication, collaboration, and community building. Part III provides tools for becoming design partners in the digital landscape and three case studies based on my own work.

The first case study describes the TangibleK robotics program for young children. It is designed as a digital playground to engage children (pre-K to second grade) and provide them with opportunities for exploring in a playful way ideas from engineering and computer science. The second case study describes a virtual world program explicitly designed for children in middle school with serious medical conditions. In this program, the Zora virtual world was designed as a multimedia park for children to build knowledge around ways to cope with their illness but also to facilitate the formation of a peer support group. The third case study presents an experience with older adolescents, incoming first-year college students, who participated in a pre-orientation program using Zora to create a campus of the future. This experience was an attempt at crafting a palace in time to explore issues of civic identity. While narrative vignettes of these three case studies can be found throughout the book, the choice here is to describe the programs in a way that isolates the elements that were considered when designing them.

This third part of the book is of particular interest to those who develop, implement, and evaluate programs that already use—or want to use—technology to promote youth development. Educators, mental health professionals, youth coordinators, program developers, and policy makers, as well as curious parents, might benefit from reading the chapters in this section. The ideas presented here can inform both formal (school-based) and informal (out-of-school) educational experiences, home-based learning, and psychotherapeutic programs, throughout the developmental span.

CHAPTER 10

Programs and Policies

When developing programs, one must be aware of the existing policies regarding children and the digital landscape, but one must also know that these policies are relatively new and are in constant flux. As new experiences are encountered, new policies are developed to address issues of public concern. Policy makers evaluate the complexities of the digital landscape and derive courses of action that attempt to balance competing interests. This happens at both the national and the federal level, at home and at school. As co-designers of the digital landscape we must be aware that it is our right and responsibility to influence the decisions that are going to affect how children experience the digital world. Sometimes, policies come to exist because of demands from the general public. These "bottom-up" initiatives can be as influential as "top-down" directives. The choice to include a brief chapter on policy in this book responds to this realization.

The first step in developing policies is to set the agenda or to identify the issue the policy will address. Once this is done, the policy can be formulated, adopted, implemented, and evaluated in an iterative cycle. In the digital landscape, policy makers have focused on how "to prohibit unfair or deceptive acts or practices in connection with the collection, use, or disclosure of personally identifiable information from and about children on the Internet." That is the agenda set forth by the Children's Online Privacy Protection Act (COPPA), which was first passed by Congress in 1998. In 2000, the Federal Trade Commission expanded on this and adopted rules to prohibit collecting personal information from children under age 13 without "verifiable parental consent" or from teachers who can act as parents' agents or intermediaries.

Most policies on the digital landscape focus on sheltering children from the risks of exposing them to adult-oriented and inappropriate content and the dangers of exploitation and abuse. At the macrolevel, COPPA protects children from giving out identifying information. However, at the microlevel of the home and school, policies also need to be put in place. Parents and teachers must discuss with their children acceptable and safe use, in a developmentally appropriate way, so that they understand the dangers of giving out age, home address, school name, or telephone number in a public forum such as chat or newsgroups. They should also agree on allowed time and duration of using a computer or any other digital device and the location of the activity.

Although sometimes it might be tempting to believe that we can create or inform policies to protect children from *all* the dangers of the digital landscape, that is not possible. As long as children inhabit and circulate in it, there will be risks, some bigger than others. Remember the playground. The best we can do is to teach children how to be "street smart" so they can better safeguard themselves in any potentially dangerous situation.

It is beyond the focus of this chapter to dwell on the safety precautions adults should take when exposing their children to the digital landscape. Much has been written on this topic, and I suggest that the interested reader consult the Child Safety on the Information Highway Web site published by the National Center for Missing and Exploited Children: http://www.safekids.com/child-safety-on-the-information-highway/.

All households should spend time setting reasonable rules and guidelines for computer use by children. Educational programs should also develop appropriate use guidelines. As children grow older, and they can engage in conversation, they should be involved in discussions to create a code of conduct for the digital landscape. This involves hard work and commitment. It is certainly tempting to install filtering software and avoid the conversation. However, as children develop technological competence and learn how the software works, they will find many creative ways to bypass it. The designer approach, where adults along with young people become active participants in developing policies for safety, fosters an open environment to address not only negative but also positive experiences in the digital landscape (Prensky, 2006).

CHAPTER 11

From Developing Curriculum to Designing Experiences

Designers of the digital landscape think about technology. However, we must avoid "technocentrism" or the natural tendency to think first about the technology and then about people and the context of its use. In my previous book, *Blocks to Robots: Learning With Technology in the Early Childhood Classroom* (Bers, 2008a), I describe how the technocentric approach often leads to a common mistake: people believe that they must first find the resources for equipping the classroom or the youth program and only then think about their educational goals and obstacles, opportunities and challenges.

Seymour Papert (1987) coined the phrase "technocentric thinking" to capture the analogy with the egocentric stage described by Piaget's developmental model of the young child. Piaget's egocentrism is not about the selfishness of the child but, rather, about his or her inability to understand anything independently of the self. Technocentrism is about to the inability of the well-intentioned educator to focus first on the human activities supported by the technology. Then, and only then, should they discuss the technology itself.

Technocentric thinking is popular among educators. After years of work, Papert warns us:

> One might imagine that "technologists" would be most likely to fall into the technocentric trap and that "humanists" would have a better understanding of the role of culture.... But things are not so simple. People from the humanities are often the most vulnerable to the technocentric trap. Insecurity sometimes makes a technical object loom too large in their thinking. Particularly in the case of computers, their intimidation and limited technical understanding often blind them to the fact that what they see as a property of "the computer" is often a cultural construct.
>
> (1987, p. 23)

When designing digital landscapes for positive youth development, we must focus on the kinds of experiences we want children to have with the technology, the kinds of activities we want them to engage in, the kinds of conversations we want them to participate in, the kinds of powerful ideas we want them to discover. the kinds of developmental opportunities we want them to encounter, and the kinds of interactions we want them to have with each other through the use of technology. Experiences happen in spaces, but these spaces, as our digital landscape shows, are not always defined by geographical location. Different types of technologies engage, encourage, and promote certain kinds of experiences while hindering others.

Experiences can be powerful because they can have an emotional impact (Brown, 2009). They transform us. They immerse us. They have an effect on our worldviews. They engage us in action. Educators have used the term *"praxis-based" models* to describe an approach for developing experiences. Praxis-based models are sometimes in sharp contrast with "knowledge-based" models. While knowledge-based models might focus on the facts, concepts, and skills that need to be taught and learned, praxis-based models look at how young people can be given opportunities for experiencing the world. Through this action-oriented process they can learn those concepts, skills, and facts.

The distinction between knowledge and praxis is consistent with the instructionist and constructionist approaches identified by Seymour Papert. The instructionist way sees the effectiveness of a technology in its instructional efficacy and, therefore, its potential for teaching, for transmitting information. In contrast, the constructionist approach conceives the computer as a tool for learners to immerse themselves in experiences that will support their own construction of knowledge. Although there is not always a clear-cut division between instructionism and constructionism, aligning instructionism with knowledge-based approaches, and constructionism with praxis-based approaches, provides a framework for thinking about the design of experiences in the digital landscape. My mentor, Seymour Papert, used to say that we "cannot think about thinking, without thinking about something." Therefore, in chapter 12 I will present three different praxis-based examples of how I have designed digital experiences for children.

Although praxis-based programs are at the heart of what I consider powerful educational experiences using technology, this view is not always in agreement with current trends in the American educational system that push for knowledge-based programs. Knowledge-based approaches are well suited to test-driven curricula; however, the metaphor of a digital landscape invites us to think beyond curriculum. We must think about experiences. We must think about immersion.

These experiences have emotional as well as cognitive, social, civic, and spiritual components.

As designers of the digital landscape, we are concerned with promoting positive youth development, and not only with improving test scores, therefore we need to take on the challenge. Some experiences happen in a natural way, for example, when children log into a Web site or play a computer game. Others happen in a structured way, by being embedded in a particular psychoeducational program (Bers, Beals, Chau, Satoh, & Khan, 2010). These experiences have clear learning goals and objectives.

Next, I will present 10 dimensions to guide the design of positive youth experiences in the digital landscape. These can be understood as questions we need to answer when conceiving these experience. They can be useful for teachers, nonformal educators, youth workers, mental health professionals, facilitators, and mentors developing these programs:

1. **Developmental milestones**: Children accomplish different developmental tasks at different ages. Using an Ericksonian framework Part 1 of the book describes this. When designing programs these developmental tasks must be considered. What are the developmental needs and milestones of the children who will be participating in this program? What are their developmental challenges? What are the developmental conflicts they are most likely to encounter?
2. **Curriculum**: The overarching goal is to design programs to support positive youth development through the affordances of the digital landscape. However, each program might also have its own unique curricular goals. What is the content, skill, or powerful idea that we want children to learn? What are the scope and sequence that should guide the teaching? Is the curriculum designed with a child-centered approach, where the agenda and pace are set by the child's interests? Is the curriculum providing a well-structured experience? What kinds of scaffolding mechanisms need to be in place?
3. **Technology**: The digital landscape offers many technologies. Each program has to make tough choices, as budget usually plays a key role. Which technologies will be used in the program? Why? What are their affordances and limitations? What needs to be in place for the technologies to be adopted in a successful way? How does the choice of technologies affect the overall experience?
4. **Mentoring model**: Designed experiences have one or multiple designers. But they also have people that carry out the designs and implement the programs. What is the role of the adults leading the program? Are they serving as coaches and mentors in the learning process? Or are they playing the role of coordinators of the experience? Are they

serving as experts? Are they taking on a teaching role? When and how should they intervene? What are the pedagogical models they will use? How many mentors should be available? What kinds of personalities and expertise should these mentors have? What kind of training should they receive?

5. **Diversity**: When using the term *diversity* we usually think in terms of ethnic, racial, religious, and socioeconomic composition. However, the fundamental diversity question we should ask in this context is: What are the diverse experiences in the digital landscape that children bring to the program? Are there shared commonalities, expectations, and needs? What kinds of diverse access to technology do children have?

6. **Program scale**: What is the size of the population we want to impact with the program? Is there a need of a minimum critical mass to sustain participants' engagement (this tends to be the case when building a social network or a virtual community)? How will self-organization, decision making, and management play out in small-scale and large-scale programs? Is there a need of institutionalization of policies? Can participants be in control of most of the decisions? If starting with a small-scale program, is there a goal to scale up? What mechanisms need to be put in place?

7. **Contact with participants**: Are participants self-selected to participate in the program? Did they go through an application process, namely, they all want and are highly motivated to participate? Is the program imposed on them? If so, what are their attitudes toward participating in the program? Is the program face-to-face, online, or a combination? If online, is the program run synchronously or asynchronously? Does the program involve regular contact among participants and with the mentors? If not, what kind of contact does it require? What are the means used for participant's contact with each other and with mentors? Is there contact with the families? In which ways?

8. **Type of assessment**: How is the program going to be evaluated? Who will conduct the evaluation? What is the goal of doing the evaluation? What elements will be considered when evaluating the program? What are the methodological approaches? Will the evaluation use ethnographic or qualitative approaches as well as quantitative ones? How will the data be collected? What are the measures of success and failure for the program?

9. **Access environment**: How are participants accessing the program? If it is an online experience, will they access from home? What elements need to be in place for successful access? What kinds of technological devices and platforms do they need? Does the experience involve both physically copresent access and online access?

10. **Institutional context**: What is the broad context in which this program will operate? What are the constraints and possibilities, opportunities and challenges, offered by the institutional context housing the program? What are the rules and policies that the program needs to adhere to?

To illustrate how each of these 10 dimensions is addressed in different experiences, I will present three case studies: a robotics program for early childhood, a virtual world intervention for late elementary and middle school children undergoing medical illness, and a pilot program for children in late adolescence who are about to start college. In each case study, the C's of the PTD framework will be highlighted, as well as their application in each unique situation.

CHAPTER 12

Case Studies

This chapter presents three case studies based on my own research. The goal is to show how the PTD framework introduced earlier has informed the design of different educational programs across the developmental span. The first case study presents an educational robotics program for early childhood, the second case study describes a virtual world program for late elementary and middle school children undergoing medical illness, and the last case study presents a pilot program for incoming college students. The design of each of the three programs is informed by the metaphors of the digital playground, the multimedia park, and the "palace in time" that were explored in the first part of this book. Instead of using a narrative approach for describing each of the experiences, each case study is organized around the 10 dimensions introduced earlier. The choice of presenting the information in that structured way is to help the reader recognize the major elements that need to be considered when purposefully designing positive experiences in the digital landscape: developmental milestones, curriculum, technology, mentoring model, diversity, project scale, contact with participants, type of assessment, access environment, and institutional context.

CASE STUDY 1: ROBOTIC PLAYGROUNDS IN EARLY CHILDHOOD

Tangible Kindergarten (TangibleK) is an early childhood robotics program that I have developed with my DevTech research team at Tufts University (Bers, 2010b). Funded by a grant from the National Science Foundation, the program engages children in learning about programming and engineering. Children participate in a curriculum that exposes them to powerful ideas from these disciplines while making robots and programming their behaviors. The TangibleK program, developed using the PTD framework, consists of a robotics curriculum, classroom assessment tools, a developmentally appropriate programming language for bringing robots to life, and a professional development component. The program has been piloted with pre-K to first grade students and teachers in the Boston area. The research done within this program shows that kindergarten-age children can understand and apply powerful computational ideas such as sequencing, control flow, sensors, loops, and branches (Bers 2007a, 2008b; Bers & Horn, 2010). Furthermore, preliminary work shows statistically significant results in terms of sequencing abilities for kindergarten students who are exposed to the TangibleK program (Kazakoff & Bers, 2011).

Using the PTD terminology, the TangibleK robotics program engages young learners in the following:

- *Content creation.* Children make robotic artifacts and program their behaviors. The engineering design process of building and the computational thinking involved in programming foster *competence* in the domains of computer literacy and technological fluency. For example, teachers who work with the TangibleK program use "engineering licenses" as a tool to assess children's levels of competence at each stage of the program. As children master a particular skill or concept, and are able to show it to a teacher, they receive a stamp on their engineering license (see Figure 12.1). These licenses are crafted following the engineering design process used for creating the robots. In similar ways as the scientific method, this iterative process gives students a tool for systematically posing a problem, doing research regarding how to address it, planning a possible solution, developing a prototype, testing the prototype, redesigning it based on findings, and sharing results with an audience that cares. Along with the engineering licenses, teachers also use design journals to scaffold the process of content creation. These journals allow children to write and draw their ideas before they go ahead in implementing them. Design journals are also used to integrate literacy activities with learning about robotics. However, while some children work best by planning in advance, others are "tinkerers" and "bricoleurs" (Turkle & Papert, 1992). They engage in negotiations with the technology; they mess around with the materials to come up with ideas. Both epistemological styles are conducive for building competence in the technological domain and are welcomed and supported in the TangibleK robotics program.
- *Creativity.* Children are invited to explore new ideas for building and programming their projects. In the TangibleK program children

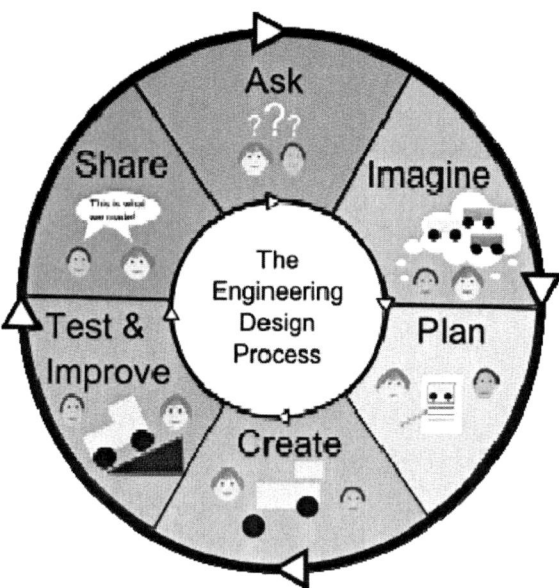

Figure 12.1. The engineering license.

explore different materials to create their robots. For example, they use LEGO pieces, motors, and sensors and integrate them with recyclable materials, arts, and crafts. The possibility of using different media engages children in exploring different approaches for their constructions. The TangibleK program is about fostering creativity, as opposed to efficiency in problem solving. However, at the end of the day, the robot will either work or not. And children will be engaged in figuring out ways to solve problems to make it work. By problem solving in creative ways, children also develop a sense of *confidence* in their learning potential. This approach is informed by the original meaning of the word *engineering*, which derives from the Latin *ingenium*, meaning "innate quality, mental power, clever invention" (*Random House Unabridged Dictionary*). Clever or creative projects involve "hard fun," a phrase used by Alan Kay (2003); they are difficult to make, time consuming, and can often lead to frustration. However, just like on the playground, children can benefit from learning how to manage frustration, an important aspect of emotional development.

- *Collaboration.* Children participate in a learning environment that promotes working in teams, sharing resources, and *caring* about each other. Most educational robotic programs for older children, such as the National Robotics Challenge and For Inspiration and Recognition of Science and Technology, are set up as competitions, events where robots have to accomplish a given task—usually outperform another robot. However, research has shown that females do not always respond well to these teaching strategies (Turbak & Berg, 2002) and that they might not be appropriate in the early childhood setting (Bers, 2008a). The TangibleK robotics program, instead of focusing on competition, promotes *caring* and working together. However, robotic technologies, unlike the Internet, do not have already built-in mechanisms to promote collaboration. Thus, we developed a low-tech tool called the "collaboration web," which is used in the classroom with this goal. The collaboration web is a personalized printout with each child's photograph in the center of the page and the photographs and names of all other children in the class arranged in a circle surrounding the main photo (see Figure 12.2). Throughout the day, each child uses the collaboration web to draw a line from his or her own photo to the photo of the children he or she had collaborated with. Here, collaboration is defined as "getting or giving help with their project, programming together, lending or borrowing materials, or working together on a common task." At the end of the week, children give out "thank-you cards" to those with whom they have collaborated the most. Depending on their abilities, children write or draw these cards. This activity is also designed to promote connections to literacy.

- *Communication.* The TangibleK program provides mechanisms to promote a sense of *connection* between peers or with adults. One of the ways the program engages students in communication is through

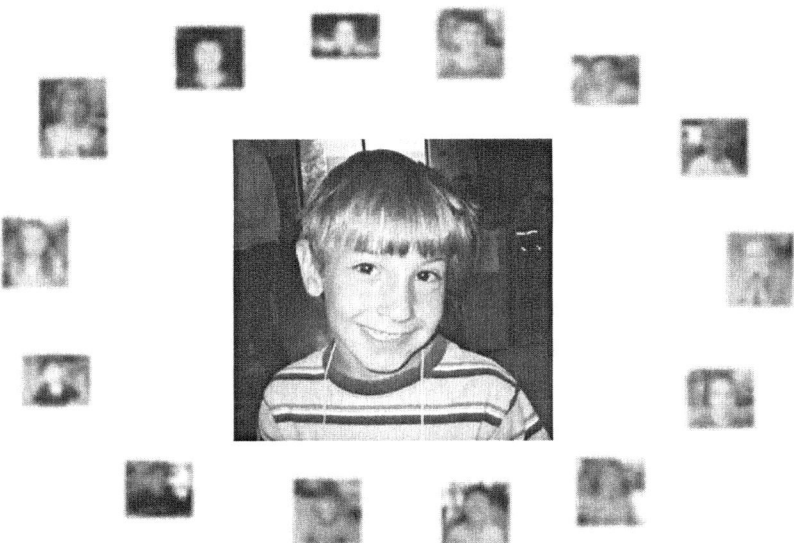

Figure 12.2. A sample collaboration web form.

technology circles—a time for all, children and adults, to stop their work, put their projects on the table or floor, sit down in a circle together, and share the state of their projects (Bers, 2008a). This is similar to other circle times in kindergarten (Kantor, Elgas, & Fernie, 1989). However, in this context, technology circles present an opportunity for debugging and solving technical problems as a community. The teacher starts the technology circle by inviting children to show their projects and asking questions such as "What worked as expected, and what didn't?" "What are you trying to accomplish?" "What do you need to know in order to make it happen?" Then, the teacher uses children's projects and questions to highlight some of the powerful ideas illustrated by the projects and to introduce new concepts. This approach provides technical information on demand, based on emerging needs, and is an alternative for lecture-style teaching. Technology circles can be called as often as every 20 minutes at the beginning of a project or only once at the end of a day of work. The decision is based on the needs of the particular group of children and the need of the teacher to introduce new concepts.

- *Community building.* Different techniques are used to scaffold the formation of a support network that *contributes* to the learning environment and community. In the spirit of the Reggio Emilia approach started by the Municipal Infant–Toddler Centers and Preschools of Reggio Emilia in Italy after World War II, projects done by children are shared with the community via an open house, demo day, or exhibition (Rinaldi, 1998). These open houses provide authentic opportunities for children to share and celebrate the process and products of their learning with others who are also invested in their learning, such as family, friends, and community members. Public displays of the learning process serve a dual function: to make learning visible to others and to the children themselves.
- *Choices of conduct.* The TangibleK program experiments with different ways to engage children in the exploration of "what if" questions and their potential consequences. This provides opportunities for children to form *character traits*. For example, children can choose to help someone who is having problems debugging her project or can choose to ignore her and continue advancing their own projects. As children make the right choices, they are given a badge by the teacher. Choices of conduct are not only made by children. Teachers make important choices in the way they display and introduce the robotic materials to the classroom. For example, if the LEGO building pieces are sorted by type and placed in bins in the center of the room (instead of giving an already sorted robotic kit to each child or group), children learn how to

take what they need without depleting the bins of the "most wanted" pieces. They also learn how to negotiate for what they need. The TangibleK program encourages teachers to think carefully about their own choices: teaching about robotics is as important as supporting children to develop an inner compass that guides their actions in a just and responsible way.

In the introduction to the book I presented a diagram with the elements of the PTD framework: (1) personal assets that are related to positive youth development (competence, confidence, character, caring, connection, and contribution), (2) positive behaviors supported by the technologies (content creation, creativity, choices of conduct, collaboration, communication, and community building), and (3) classroom practice. This third column refers to how each particular educational program conceives mechanisms to support the work with technology in a way that fits with its own learning culture, rituals, and values. In the PTD diagram presented earlier it was left blank. This was done purposefully. In the early part of this book I introduced PTD as an abstract framework that could inform the design of any educational program. However, here I will present how PTD informs a particular program: TangibleK. Thus, the same graphic will be shown again, but this time with the third column completed with information relevant to the practices of the TangibleK program (see Figure 12.3).

DESIGN DIMENSIONS

While a significant amount of research focuses on robotics education for middle school and high school as well as college, little work is focused in the foundational years (Bers, 2008a; Rogers & Portsmore, 2004). We know, however, from both an economic and a developmental standpoint, that educational interventions that begin in early childhood are associated with lower costs and stronger, more durable effects than interventions that begin later in childhood (Cunha & Heckman, 2006; Heckman & Masterov, 2004).

For decades the early childhood curriculum has focused on literacy and numeracy, with some attention paid to the natural sciences. However, in today's world technology and engineering, the missing "T" and "E" of STEM—science, technology, engineering, and mathematics—education in early childhood, play an important role. In my previous book, *Blocks to Robots: Learning With Technology in the Early Childhood Classroom* (Bers, 2008a), I have explored this in depth.

(146) Plotting learning trajectories through design

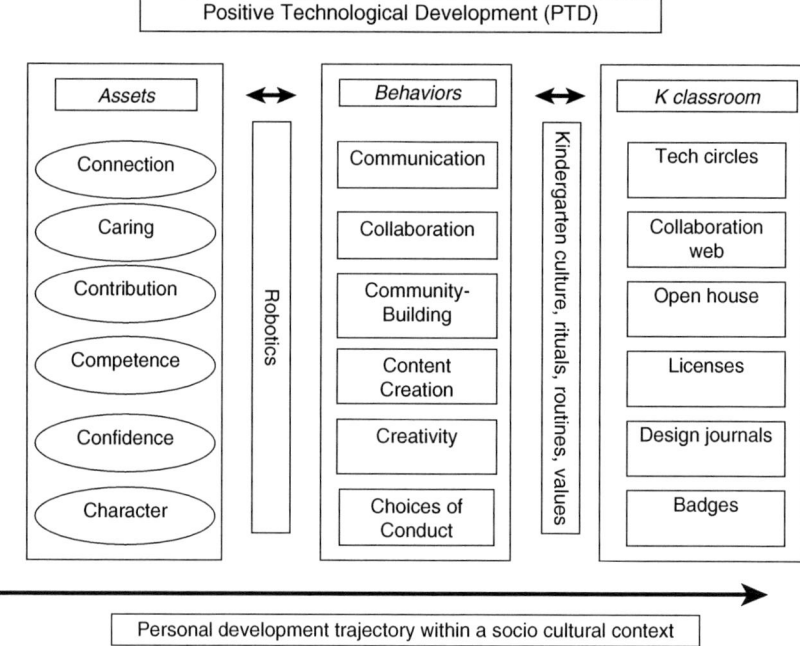

Figure 12.3. The PTD framework as it informs the practice in a kindergarten robotics program.

The need to expose young children to experiences that support knowledge of the surrounding human-made world motivated the TangibleK project. In the following paragraphs, the program is described around the 10 dimensions presented earlier.

1. Developmental Milestones

The program is explicitly designed for children in the age range of four to seven years old. A child who is in pre-K to first grade is likely to be transitioning between the Piagetian preoperational stage, when she is not yet able to think abstractly and needs concrete physical objects, and the concrete operational stage, when she starts to conceptualize abstractions, creating logical structures that explain her physical experiences. This is a period when children might not read and write yet, although they have mastered the use of spoken language. In terms of social development, they are learning to work cooperatively and have a difficult time seeing things from another's point of view. Children depend on authority and like rules and routines. They benefit from both structured predictable schedules and exploratory time to experiment on their own. Erikson's psychosocial theory situates children in this age range as negotiating *initiative vs. guilt*, with the resulting virtue or developmental milestone being a sense of accomplishment for intentionally doing something—for example, making and programming a robot that accomplishes a task.

2. Curriculum

The TangibleK curriculum introduces powerful ideas from computer science in a robotics context in a structured, developmentally appropriate way. The term *powerful idea* refers to a central concept within a domain that is at once epistemologically and personally useful, interconnected with other disciplines, and has roots in intuitive knowledge that a child has internalized over a long period of time (Bers, Ponte, et al., 2002; Papert, 1980). The powerful ideas addressed in this curriculum include robotics, the engineering design process, sequencing and control flow, loops and parameters, and sensors and branches. Table 12.1 describes

Table 12.1. POWERFUL IDEAS, DEFINITIONS, ACTIVITIES, AND INTERDISCIPLINARY CONNECTIONS OF THE TANGIBLEK PROGRAM

Powerful Idea	Definition	Activity	Discipline Connections
Robotics	The engineering discipline that focuses on the creation and programming of robots, machines that can follow instructions and move on their own to perform tasks.	*What Is a Robot?* After an introduction to robotics by looking at different robots and talking about the functions they serve, children build their own robotic vehicles and explore their parts and the instructions they can use to program them.	Engineering Computer science
Engineering design process	A process used to develop products to solve a need or problem. It has several iterative steps: identifying a need or defining the problem, doing research, analyzing possible solutions, developing the product, communicating and presenting the product.	*Sturdy Building*: Children build a nonrobotic vehicle to take small toy people from home to school. The vehicle needs to be sturdy as well as perform its intended functions. *Design Journals*: Children use the design journals to document the process.	Engineering Computer science

(Continued)

Table 12.1. (CONTINUED)

Powerful Idea	Definition	Activity	Discipline Connections
Sequencing/ control flow	A sequence of instructions can be described in a program and acted out in order by a robot. Each block has a specific meaning. The order of the blocks is important.	*The Hokey Pokey*: Children choose the appropriate commands and put them in order to program a robot to dance the hokey pokey.	Creative storytelling Organization of ideas Mathematical proofs Procedural thinking
Loops and parameters	A sequence of instructions can be modified to occur over and over again. This sequence can be qualified with additional information. For example, loops can repeat forever or for a concrete number of times.	*Again and Again Until I Say When*: Children use a pair of loop blocks ("repeat"/"end repeat") to make the robot go forward again and again, infinitely, and then just the right number of times to arrive at a fixed location.	Cyclical events in nature Scheduling Timing and control Feedback loops Number sense
Sensors	A robot can use sensors, akin to human sense organs, to gather information from its environment. Sensors information can control when the robot follows given commands.	*Through the Tunnel*: Children use light sensors and commands to program a robot to turn its lights on when its surroundings are dark and vice versa.	Scientific observations Cause and effect Sensors (both human-made and natural)
Branches	At a branch in the program, a robot can follow one set of commands or another depending on the state of a given condition.	*The Robot Decides*: Students program their robot to travel to one of two destinations based on light or touch sensor information.	Cause and effect Sensors (human-made and natural)

these concepts and shows the specific activities done in the curriculum, as well as the interdisciplinary connections. While the powerful ideas remain the same, different versions of the curriculum apply them to different themes, such as transportation, community, animals, and exploration of identity (Bers, 2010b).

The curriculum has six structured lessons focusing on powerful ideas and an open thematic block at the end for students to apply the gained knowledge and skills to their own personally meaningful projects. Depending on the classroom and the time the teacher can devote to the

TangibleK program, each lesson might take as little as one hour or span several hours of classroom work. The same happens for the open thematic block. Each of the six lessons in the curriculum has learning objectives defined in terms of both what the students should understand and what they should be able to do (see Table 12.2).

In previous work, during the open thematic block, children created a robotic city, a zoo with animals that moved, a route map for snowplows to travel from children's homes to school, a dinosaur park, and a garden with robotic flowers responsive to different sensors (Bers, 2008a). They have

Table 12.2. LEARNING OBJECTIVES FOR EACH OF THE SIX LESSONS

Lesson	Students will understand that...	Students will be able to...
1. Sturdy building (engineering design process)	• LEGO bricks and other materials can fit together to form sturdy structures. • The engineering design process is useful for planning and guiding the creation of artifacts.	• Build a sturdy, nonrobotic vehicle using LEGO bricks and other materials. • Use design journals to learn the engineering design process.
2. What is a robot? (robots have special parts to follow instructions)	• Robots need moving parts, such as motors, to be able to perform behaviors specified by a program. • The robotic brain has the programmed instructions that make the robot perform its behaviors. • The robotic brain must communicate with the motors for the motors to function.	• Describe the components of a robot, including the robotic brain, motors, and wires. • Upload a program to a robot via the tangible blocks or graphical icons, computer interface, and LEGO tower. • Build a sturdy, robotic vehicle using LEGO bricks and other materials.
3. Hockey Pokey (sequence of commands matters)	• Each icon corresponds to a specific command. • A program is a sequence of commands that is followed by a robot. • The order of the blocks dictates the order in which the robot executes the commands.	• Select the appropriate block corresponding to a planned robot action. • Connect a series of blocks. • Upload a program to the computer and transmit it to a robot.
4. Again and Again Until I Say When (loops and number parameters)	• A command or sequence of commands may be modified to repeat. • Some programming commands, like "Repeat," can be modified with additional information. • A simple program that uses fewer blocks is better than a more complex one that accomplishes the same goal.	• Recognize a situation that requires a program to use loops. • Write a program that loops. • Use parameters to modify the number of times a loop runs before the program stops.

(Continued)

Table 12.2. (CONTINUED)

Lesson	Students will understand that...	Students will be able to...
5. Through the Tunnel (sensors and loops)	• Through the use of sensors, a robot can feel and see its surroundings. • A robot can react to collected data by changing its behavior. • A robot can be programmed to remain on a certain task until a specific condition is met.	• Connect a light or touch sensor to the correct port on the robotic brain. • Write a program that includes waiting for a specific condition.
6. The Robot Decides (sensors and branches)	• A robot can "choose" between two sequences of commands depending on the state of a given condition.	• Connect a sensor to the correct port on the robot. • Identify a situation that calls for a branched program. • Write a program that uses a branch.

also explored issues of identity such as the "Mi Ani?" (Who am I?) project, which engaged children in building a robot that would represent them traveling through the different Jewish and secular holidays during the year (Libman, 2011). All of these final projects used inexpensive recyclable materials and arts and crafts, as well the robotic components. For example, one kindergarten classroom in Boston, after taking a field trip to the old city, constructed a robotic Freedom Trail, using cardboard boxes to re-create the historical buildings of the city and embedding light sensors and motors into the boxes to bring the buildings to life (Bers, 2008a).

3. Technology

The choice of technology for the TangibleK program is based upon the research-based evidence collected over more than 16 years of working with young children and robotics (Bers, 2008a, 2008b; Cejka, Rogers, & Portsmore, 2006). Over those years, I have worked with diverse prototypes developed both at the MIT Media Lab (Martin et al., 2000) and at Tufts University (Rogers & Portsmore, 2004) and commercially available robotic kits developed by the LEGO company. However, none of those has a developmentally appropriate interface for young children. With funding from the National Science Foundation, my research team developed a system, the Creative Hybrid Environment for Robotic Programming, that allows young children to program with interlocking

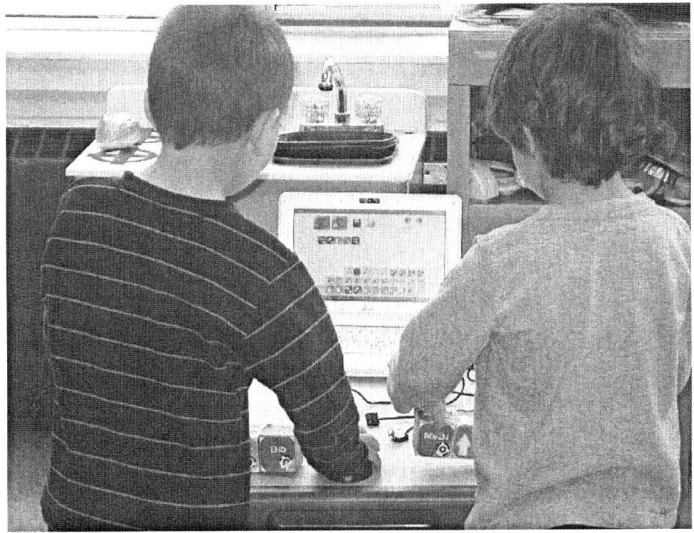

Figure 12.4. The CHERP language developed at Tufts University. Children construct programs for their robots using interlocking wooden blocks.

wooden blocks (see Figure 12.4) and to transition back and forth between the screen-based and the tangible programming language (Bers & Horn, 2010). This hybrid approach allows children to work with multiple representations, in the same way that they learn math or literacy by using different media (Horn et al., 2011).

CHERP uses a collection of image-processing techniques to convert physical programs into digital instructions (Horn & Jacob, 2007; Horn et al., 2011). Each block in the language is imprinted with a circular symbol called a TopCode. These codes allow the position, orientation, size, shape, and type of each block to be quickly determined from a digital image. A standard Webcam connected to a desktop or laptop computer takes a picture of the program. A compiler converts the picture into digital code, which gets downloaded to the robot in a matter of seconds (see Figure 12.5).

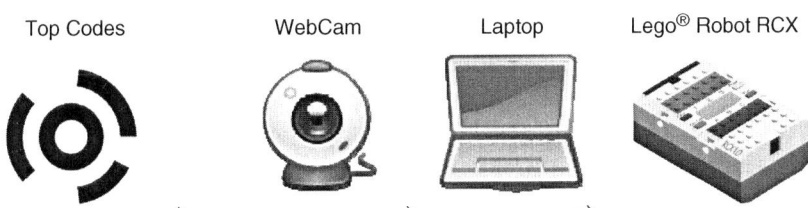

Figure 12.5. The download process.

As shown in Figure 12.5, the programs children create with CHERP can be downloaded to the LEGO RCX brick, an embedded microcomputer or the "robot brain," contained in the LEGO MINDSTORMS kit. We are currently exploring the use of other robotic kits that might provide a cheaper alternative. However, discussing these technical options is beyond the scope of this chapter.

4. Mentoring Model

The TangibleK program engages kindergarten teachers in their traditional roles. One of the program successes is that it does not impose a foreign teaching model but, rather, draws from existing practices in the kindergarten classroom. However, it pushes teachers out of their comfort zone by using robotics. For that purpose, participating teachers are required to attend professional development. For the program to run smoothly in the classroom there is need of a high ratio of adults to children. It is recommended to have a minimum of one adult for every 10 students. The role of these adults is to help children manipulate their robotic artifacts, set up the computers, and provide on-demand help to children who have questions as they work on their own projects. Depending on the classroom, helpers can be volunteer parents and grandparents, preservice teachers doing their training, or graduate students and children in older grades who are assigned buddies in the kindergarten classroom.

5. Diversity

Kindergarten children come to school with diverse exposure to and experience working with computers and building with LEGO bricks. While some are very familiar with the mouse and keyboard and can navigate the desktop interface with ease, others have a difficult time. These differences are taken into consideration before engaging children in the TangibleK program. Ideally teachers can plan ahead and slowly integrate the use of computers and LEGO bricks into their elective activities and choice time.

6. Program Scale

The TangibleK program is aimed at prekindergarten to second grade classrooms. Thus, the size of the program varies according to the class size—usually ranging between 16 and 24 children. When several classes in the same school want to participate in the program at the same time, there are advantages and disadvantages. On the positive side, teachers become a learning community and can provide help and support to each other. On the negative side, the school needs to have more available technological resources or coordinate staggering the work among classrooms, as it is not always possible to disassemble the robotic creations on time for a new group.

7. Contact With Participants

The TangibleK program is designed for a minimum of 20 hours of classroom work, divided into six structured sessions, based on the powerful ideas presented earlier, and the open thematic block. These hours can be spread over several months or can be condensed into an intensive and immersive experience. Each session follows a similar structure: (1) warm-up games to introduce the powerful idea in a playful way, (2) a building and/or programming task to reinforce the powerful idea, (3) individual or pairs work on a small project to put to use the powerful idea in a new context, (4) a technology circle to debrief and reinforce the concept, and (5) assessment. After six sessions, in which teachers introduce powerful ideas and children can experiment with them through structured tasks, it is time for the open thematic block. This is an opportunity for students to revisit the learned concepts and skills but to apply them to a project of their own choice. The length of time assigned to these projects varies according to the classroom and to the teachers' goals and expectations, as well as to the curricular demands. These final projects are shared in an open house with the wider community.

8. Type of Assessment

The PTD framework guides the program evaluation. Thus, teaching about robotics is as important as helping the child develop in an integrated and holistic way. The assessment is not limited to the cognitive dimension. The TangibleK program extends its efforts for evaluation to the social and the moral dimensions of the child's experience through and with the technology.

The first two C's, *content creation* and *creativity*, are evaluated in terms of competence (or level of understanding) and confidence in the domain of robotics and computer programming. The following tools and techniques are used to assess these two C's:

a. Student portfolios: These are composed of students' design journals, students' programming samples (code), and students' robotic projects. Change over time in the level of sophistication and complexity is assessed.
b. Video journals: Children are videotaped showing what they have been working on and explaining their doings at least at three points in time in the program (e.g., beginning, middle, and end).
c. Rubric of levels of understanding: This consists of a set of questions for the teacher or researcher to complete at the end of each session aimed at assessing the level of understanding of each child on a scale of 0 to 5, for each of the learning objectives throughout the curriculum and for each of the tasks at different levels of complexity. Table 12.3 is an example of the assessment rubric for session 2, which engages children in programming their robot to dance the hokey pokey and introduces the powerful idea of "the order or sequence of instructions matters," a key concept in computational thinking.

Table 12.3. RUBRIC OF LEVELS OF UNDERSTANDING

Part 1: Circle the corresponding level of achievement for each child for each statement listed. Circle NA if the statement could not be assessed during this activity.

5	4	3	2	1	0
Achieves without assistance	Achieves with minimal assistance	Achieves with periodic assistance	Achieves with significant assistance	Achieves with step-by-step instructions	Does not achieve

1. A. Works purposefully toward the goal of the activity.	5 4 3 2 1 0 NA
1. B. Works purposefully toward self-selected goal. If so, what goal?	5 4 3 2 1 0 NA
2. If working on a self-selected goal, he or she can articulate the goal.	5 4 3 2 1 0 NA
3. Translates his or her ideas into code for the robot to act out.	5 4 3 2 1 0 NA
4. Arranges blocks or icons in a syntactically correct sequence to make a functional program.	5 4 3 2 1 0 NA
5. A. Recognizes incorrect actions or order in a program by reading the program or watching the robot run the program.	5 4 3 2 1 0 NA
5. B. Has a hypothesis of the problem.	5 4 3 2 1 0 NA
5. C. Attempts to solve the problem	5 4 3 2 1 0 NA
6. Selects correct instructions for the program based on their corresponding actions.	5 4 3 2 1 0 NA
7. Robot maintains its core integrity while being handled and while it runs programs.	5 4 3 2 1 0 NA
8. Understands that programs made in the TUI and GUI must be translated and sent to the robot by the computer.	5 4 3 2 1 0 NA

Table 12.3. (CONTINUED)

Part 2: Ask each child questions such as "When you make a program, does it make a difference what order you put the blocks in?" to supplement the students' journals and the teachers' observations of and conversations with students during work and sharing times. Mark the students' level of understanding of how to program a robot along the following criteria.

Syntactic:	Understands the function of individual instructions but not how to choose and assemble them to make a functional program that accomplishes a given goal.
Semantic:	Chooses appropriate instructions for the program and puts them in the right order. Understands that putting the parts together in certain ways creates an overall outcome. May not be able to create a program that completely meets the given goal or may not realize it when the goal is met.
Systems:	Understands the function of each element and that the order they are put in results in a specific overall outcome. Is able to purposefully put the right instructions in the right order for the program to achieve the given goal.

The other two C's, *collaboration* and *communication*, are evaluated in terms of the levels of caring and connection achieved by the children by analyzing the collaboration webs over time and children's participation in the technology circles. The last C's, *community building* and *choices of conduct*, are evaluated by looking at the child's overall participation and engagement in the TangibleK program and her *contributions* to the learning environment, in particular through the lens of the final project presented at the open house and the earned expertise badges as representatives of the child's character traits. Change over time is analyzed.

9. Access Environment

The TangibleK program runs in classrooms located within schools. Based on the particular goals and capabilities of each classroom, it will be decided how many children will work together in the same group or if children will work individually. The essential elements for a school to successfully run this program are to have the available technology, trained staff and institutional support for professional development, and scheduling flexibility.

10. Institutional Context

The TangibleK program can be adapted to work in different institutional contexts, as long as teachers have the flexibility to incorporate a new area of study, such as robotics and programming, into their curriculum. The institution needs to support the purchase of equipment and the staff release time to participate in professional development.

CASE STUDY 2: VIRTUAL WORLDS FOR MEDICALLY ILL PEDIATRIC PATIENTS

This case study describes the innovative use of the Zora virtual world in two interventions for children with critical medical conditions. The first one involves post-transplant youth from two different hospitals. They used Zora from their homes to address issues of medical adherence and school transition in the context of a peer-support network (Bers, 2009; Bers, Beals, Chau, Satoh, Blume, et al., 2010). The second case involves a group of youth with cancer and sickle cell and healthy siblings participating in Camp for All in Burton, Texas, a summer camp for ill children and their families (Cantrell & Bers, 2010; Cantrell, Fischer, Bouzaher, & Bers, 2010). Children participating in both of these experiences were in middle school.

Using the PTD terminology, the Zora program engages pediatric patients in the following:

- *Content creation.* Children build their virtual homes and public spaces of interest, decorating them with pictures and writing stories about their experiences. Children also program interactive characters, such as favorite doctors, to engage with them in conversations and hear their stories. Zora provides authoring tools that promote *competence* in the development of technological fluency. For example, children created interactive objects to express issues of school transition and games to share strategies for completing homework while in the hospital. They also created a "Health Museum" to display their own medical stories and a "Hope Hut" to share hopeful memories related to illness.
- *Creativity.* Children use different media in Zora to express their fears, feelings, and fantasies. For example, participants collaboratively built a Halloween house where they posted stories about "the things they were most afraid of," a Zora restaurant with menus displaying the "forbidden food that you can eat in a virtual world," and a pharmacy to learn strategies for remembering to take their medicines. They also created a "Legislature House" where they wrote recommendations for hospitals to ease the stay of the patients, such as "soft pillows, beds with comfortable mattress pads on them . . . especially in the cardiac cathlab, where

you have to lay flat for six hours," and suggestions for schools to ease transitions after prolonged hospitalizations. While creating these online projects, children develop a sense of *confidence* in their creative potential and their sense of pride as learners grows. This is particularly important for those children who cannot attend school on a regular basis.

- *Collaboration.* Children worked together on virtual projects and supported each other in different *caring* ways. While Zora has tools for participants to work individually, virtual group activities successfully bring the community together. For example, every month the virtual community comes together to produce a newsletter (the post-transplant group voted to call it *Transplant Times*). Children take on the roles of writers, interviewers, and photographers to report their experiences and activities in Zora. The newsletter is printed out and distributed to families and physicians as a way to share participants' experiences. For example, children interviewed a physician who came to Zora as a guest and a first-year student in college who'd had a transplant and shared advice about coping with medical illness leaving home.

- *Communication.* Zora offers both synchronous and asynchronous ways of communication, which promote a sense of *connection* between peers or with adults. Participants communicate about health-related issues but also share their needs, feelings, and worries. A social worker described Zora as providing "something that none of [the patient's] Doctors or medical professionals could—a connection to other kids who knew exactly how he was feeling and experience the unpleasant things that go along with transplant each and every day." While most participants benefit from an online peer community, others seek to extend their new friendships to offline activities. For example, two female transplant recipients reported that Zora helped them meet each other for the first time, but then, once they had established an online friendship, they chose to continue meeting face-to-face.

- *Community building.* Zora offers spaces and tools that enable the formation of a social support network that can expand, in some cases, to face-to-face exchanges. This promotes *contribution* to the Zora community and beyond. For example, a 15-year-old female post–liver transplant patient wrote in Zora:

> I believe that taking part in Zora did give me inspiration. I only had a liver transplant, and I cannot have tunnel vision that there's only me, but there are a multitude of other kids that have gone through similar experiences as myself. They inspired me to help educate others about organ donation, because there are kids like us whose lives have been saved through the gift of organ donation.

As a result of her participation in Zora, this girl made a PowerPoint presentation to teach her school classmates about organ transplantation and organ donation. Back in Zora she created a virtual information booth where she linked her presentation so that other Zora children could borrow it and advocate in their own schools. A different type of community-building event happened at the end of the year, when a Zora group and their families decided to participate in the hospital's annual fundraising walk. This was the first time they met each other face-to-face.

- *Choices of conduct.* Zora has features explicitly designed to support users to explore *character traits* and their ethical and moral values. For example, children can use the collaborative values dictionary to create their own values and discuss how to create a safe environment for everyone. They can also make models of identification, such as heroes and villains.

In the book's introduction I presented the PTD diagram with empty boxes in the concrete practices column. In the previous section, I showed the completed graphic based on the TangibleK program. In Figure 12.6,

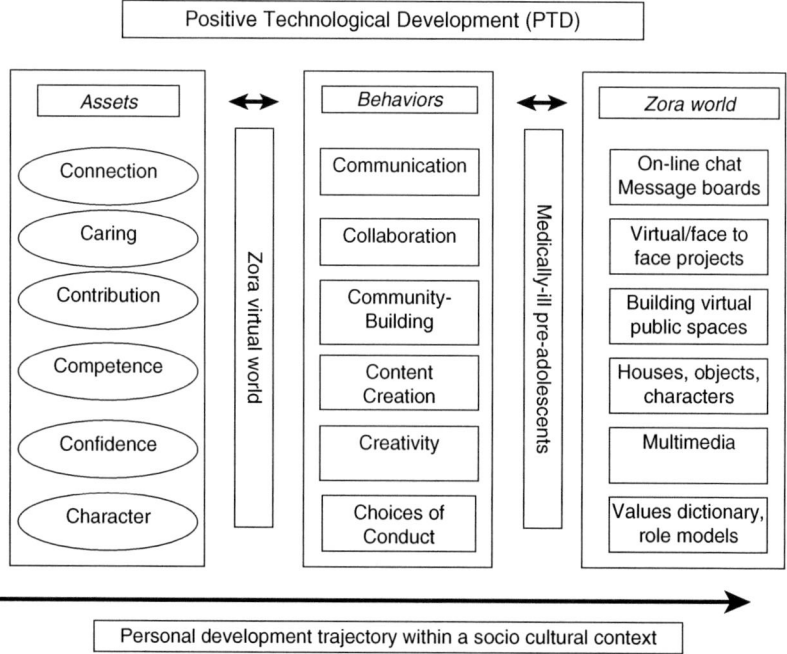

Figure 12.6. The PTD framework as it informs the practice in the Zora virtual world for medically ill children.

I present it one more time with the practices of the Zora program for medically ill children. Since Zora was explicitly designed following the PTD framework, there is alignment between the affordances of the technology and the positive behaviors and practices it supports.

My research team and colleagues conducted different pilot studies with preadolescents facing serious medical illness. The first study, in collaboration with pediatric psychiatrists and medical staff in the pediatric transplant program at Boston Children's Hospital and the Tufts Floating Hospital for Children, had the goals to facilitate peer networking, encourage medical adherence through online activities, and support patients' psychosocial adjustment to school transition and lifestyle changes. Most participants used Zora from their homes and, at times, during hospitalizations (Bers, Beals, Chau, Satoh, Blume, et al., 2010; Bers, Beals, Chau, Satoh, & Khan, 2010; Bers et al., 2007).

The second pilot study involved the use of Zora in the context of a summer camp in Texas for children with cancer and blood disorders and their healthy siblings (Cantrell & Bers, 2010). The goal of the program was to explore if participation in Zora after the end of the week of camp could sustain the campers' hopefulness and sense of connectedness achieved during camp.

DESIGN DIMENSIONS

As young people discover new ways of using the Internet for social interaction, graphical virtual worlds are emerging as one of the fastest growing online environments for youth (Beals & Bers, 2009). Virtual worlds' psychosocial interventions provide a wonderful opportunity to reach children who, due to geographical distance, cannot attend face-to-face meetings (Bers, Beals, Chau, Satoh, Blume, et al., 2010).

In the past, most young people with a serious medical illness would not survive. Today, advances in medicine make it possible to extend the length of their lives. However, children are trading a life-limiting disease for invasive follow-up interventions and the hardships of medical adherence associated with difficulties in transitioning back to school and socially engaging with peers (Griffin & Elkin, 2001). Frequent clinic visits, medication intake, and dietary and physical exercise restrictions can be disruptive to the patients' academic and social life (Brem, Brem, McGrath, & Spirito, 1988; Erikson, 1950; Gerson, Furth, Neu, & Fivush, 2004; Rodin & Voshart, 1987). Therefore it is crucial that help is provided to address the medical, psychosocial, educational, and vocational needs of the patients at various stages of their lives (Engle, 2001). Unfortunately, psychosocial services lag behind medical advances, as it is difficult to run effective programs for patients who are geographically dispersed and small in number. Thus, there is a need to find other vehicles through which to provide the needed supports. This is the driving force of the Zora virtual world programs described in this section.

1. Developmental Milestones

Preadolescence stands between the security and safety of childhood and the freedom and responsibilities of adolescence. The lives of preadolescents are centered around peer friendships, school, and after-school activities. According to Erikson's theory, preadolescents are busy developing a sense of industry by gaining new skills and knowledge and at the same time might experience unresolved feelings of inadequacy and inferiority among their peers. Unlike for adolescents, identity development is not yet a major developmental task; however, preadolescents are starting to explore their role as unique individuals distinct from their own families and as members of peer groups, if not yet the wider society (Berk, 2008; Rubin, Bukowski, & Parker, 2006). Laura Beals's dissertation explores the role of virtual worlds in supporting preadolescents' development. She (2011) writes that two changes are important to virtual worlds during these stages: (1) the improvement of spatial reasoning, which includes the ability to give directions and to draw and read maps, and (2) a decrease in egocentrism, which allows children to communicate about objects that others cannot see and to consider the perspectives of another.

2. Curriculum

The Zora curriculum is made up of six objectives that mirror the six C's of PTD. Throughout the virtual experience, participants are encouraged to complete the objectives within the curriculum at their own pace. While synchronous online meetings allow children to come together, the curriculum follows a loose structure and sequence to encourage and accommodate differentiated access, levels of instruction, time zones, and previous expertise. Zora mentors keep track of the youth's progress through the curricular activities. When a child comes online, the mentors assist her on an individual basis, matching the learning to her progress. Table 12.4 briefly describes each of the six objectives within the curriculum and provides a sample Zora activity to address issues of school transition. Overall, during the eight-month post-transplant study, users created a total of 4,027 objects and made 75 virtual houses.

Table 12.4. CURRICULUM CHART

Objective	PTD	PYD	Sample Activity (Prompt to Child)	Relevance
1	Content Creation	Competence	Construct a virtual object that represents a struggle you face while at school.	Communication with educators and families is crucial. Objective 1 promotes communication about school issues.
2	Creativity	Confidence	Construct a virtual space with objects that represent solutions to the school struggle.	Objective 2 promotes initiative and problem solving related to school transition.
3	Collaboration	Caring	Interview another participant about his or her school struggles and school solutions objects.	Objective 3 promotes awareness of the many school transition concerns.
4	Communication	Connection	Make and program an interactive character that represents someone who has helped you through your transplant experience.	Objective 4 promotes communication about the importance of proper medical care and its continuation through adherence.
5	Community building	Contribution	Participate in the virtual scavenger hunt and reflect on the experience within Zora. How has it helped you?	Objective 5 encourages reflection on the community composed of fellow transplant recipients.
6	Choice of Conduct	Character	Construct an innovative virtual object that will help you manage your medical routine. Add a value for this object and define it.	Objective 6 encourages independent consideration of adherence and creative problem solving related to medical regime. It also promotes adherence responsibility.

3. Technology

Zora is a 3-D virtual environment with easy-to-use authoring tools. I designed the first version of Zora in 1999 using the Microsoft Virtual Worlds development platform, as part of my doctoral work at MIT (Bers, 2001). The current version of Zora used in the studies described in this chapter has been updated and extended using the ActiveWorlds platform (Bers, 2007b; Satoh, McVey, Grogan, & Bers, 2006). Users interact and communicate with each other in real time through a chat system, as well as in asynchronous ways through message boards. Users are graphically represented as avatars. They can populate the virtual world with their own interactive creations by designing 3-D graphical objects, interactive characters that can hold "conversations" with visitors, and personal and public spaces. Although Zora provides authoring tools, the focus is not on the aesthetics of the 3-D objects but, rather, on the meanings assigned to them. Thus the design elements of Zora encourage users to create stories and values for every object they make in the world, models of identification (such as heroes and villains) for their avatar profiles, and a collective values dictionary for the resulting virtual community. In Zora youth engage in chatting as well as doing, discussing as well as creating, thinking as well as producing (Bers, Beals, Chau, Satoh, & Khan, 2010). Zora has similarities with the growingly popular Second Life virtual world (Ondrejka, 2004) in presenting a three-dimensional environment for users to develop a virtual community. However, unlike Second Life, Zora is a secured and password-protected world in which only youth with a particular educational program or intervention can view and access the world and contribute to it. For example, in the summer camp program, the Zora world was designed to mirror the actual physical campsite, with the dining hall and the cabins, a virtual lake, and areas for the various activities offered at camp such as a ropes course and horses (see Figure 12.7). Zora was explicitly designed following the PTD framework

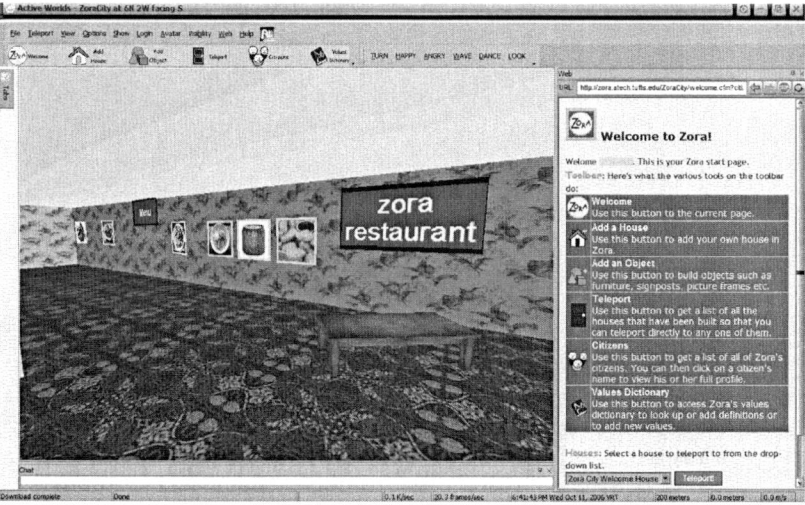

Figure 12.7. Image of the Zora virtual world including chat bar (bottom), navigation screen (middle), and welcome screen (right).

(Bers, 2006). Thus, it supports the implementation of a virtual curriculum that takes advantage of the features of Zora that are well aligned with the theoretical model.

4. Mentoring Model

The mentoring model in the Zora program is composed of a facilitator with experience in child health and pediatric psychology, and a clear agenda in terms of the research and learning goals of the project, and several e-mentors. The facilitator coordinates weekly Zora online activities, and the e-mentors provide technical help and support (Cantrell et al., 2010). In addition, depending on the group, older teenagers who had a transplant or who were camp leaders were identified as mentors for the Zora community and were invited to join.

5. Diversity

The diversity among participants is found in terms of the type of medical illness, the type of organ they received, the types of medical situations that led them to require an organ transplant, the time since transplant, and the severity of their condition. Diversity is also found in terms of geographical location and home-based hospital, as children participating in the studies came from several states across the United States, and diverse socioeconomic status and ethnicity.

6. Project Scale

The Zora programs described here were of small scale. For example, in the post-transplant study, although 32 post-transplant patients signed consent forms, only 21 used Zora. At the beginning of the project the small scale was not an issue, and children were happy to meet other post-transplant children for the first time. However, as the project evolved, children wanted more participants, as it was difficult to have synchronous activities and conversations. Throughout the study, we held weekly online meetings at two different times to accommodate schedules and time zones. In addition, the voluntary nature of the project meant that we could not enforce regular attendance. Thus sometimes as few as one or two participants attended planned activities. However, participants would be online at other times to work on individual projects. Due to the "constant on" nature of this project, participants were welcomed to sign on at any time; however, our data showed that in many cases, a participant who logged on and found that only one or two other members were on would sign off. This is consistent with research that shows the importance of a minimum critical mass to sustain participants' engagement when building a social network or a virtual community (e.g., Markus, 1987; Preece, 2000). During the camp experience, although 40 campers signed consent forms, only 19 used Zora, and only 10 participated weekly, completing the entire curriculum.

7. Types of Contact With Participants

Most contact with participants happened online, except before the start of the program when parents and children had to sign consent forms. In both studies, e-mail became the most reliable tool for communicating with the families, and updates came nearly daily. In addition to logistical and scheduling e-mails, interviews with the participants were done. During the post-transplant study each user logged into Zora an average of 60 times and spent an average of 39 hours logged into the program. This represents almost seven hours more online time than we had anticipated, as we had planned weekly online activities for 32 hours (Bers, Beals, Chau, Satoh, Blume, et al., 2010). During the course of the study, three individuals underwent cardiac re-transplantation. Their participation from the hospital both before and after the transplant added an extra dimension to group discussions. It also provided an opportunity for some of the participants to meet face-to-face. Based on computer log analysis, it became clear that patients with high severity in their illness were the ones who used Zora the most (Bers, Beals, Chau, Satoh, Blume, et al., 2010).

8. Type of Assessment

Data collection included automatically generated computer logs that provide qualitative and quantitative data of users' online activities, self-report instruments, and semistructured interviews, as well as spontaneous feedback. Data about patients' medical adherence and medical history were provided by parents, medical staff, and children themselves. During the camp experience, data collection was conducted in two phases. The first phase was at camp, face-to-face while the campers were introduced to the Zora program. The second phase of data collection occurred over the phone after six weeks of program usage.

9. Access Environment

The participants were expected to log online from their home computers. Thanks to a grant from the National Science Foundation, we were able to provide free access to a computer suitable for using Zora and free Internet service for the duration of the study to post-transplant children who needed it. During hospitalizations, patients accessed Zora from the hospital. During the camp experience, computers were used at camp, and later a CD was provided to all participants who assented so that they could install Zora back at home and continue using the program. Additionally, the two participating hospitals installed the program on their computers.

10. Institutional Context of Usage

Participants were requested to sign a Code of Conduct outlining basic rules of Internet behavior (such as not disclosing personal information online) prior to logging into Zora for the first time. This was in accordance with hospital regulations. During the camp experience, the Code of Conduct mirrored many of the ethical codes established at Camp for All. In both programs, the initial items on the Code of Conduct were created by the research team, but once on Zora, children were encouraged to discuss appropriate and inappropriate behavior. Once consensus was reached as a community, new items were added to the Code of Conduct in the Zora world. In both studies, the program strictly adhered to Institutional Review Board recommendations, such as daily monitoring of online logs and a reporting system in case the facilitator or mentors encountered problematic content.

CASE STUDY 3: A COLLEGE CAMPUS OF THE FUTURE

Active Citizenship Through Technology (ACT) was a pilot pre-orientation program for incoming college students at Tufts University conducted with funding from Tisch College. The program was held first in 2006 and then again in 2007 (Bers, 2008a, 2008c; Bers & Chau, 2010). ACT engages students in civic dialogue early in their academic experience while fostering a long-term peer support network. It leverages youth's interest in the digital landscape to engage them in civic discussions and activities. In this three-day program, participants use Zora to design and inhabit a virtual campus of the future to express concerns and ideas about community issues of interest. In addition, they participate in face-to-face activities to promote civic skills and learn about their college community.

Using the PTD terminology, the ACT program engages incoming first-year students in the following:

- *Content creation.* Zora provides tools to create a campus of the future with virtual spaces representing personal and civic interests. In the process, students develop technological *competence*. Throughout the ACT program, students used Zora to graphically display information gathered from visits around campus and the surrounding neighborhoods in the form of 3-D virtual exhibits. Participants interviewed members of academic departments and key leaders on campus and in the local community and went back to the Zora world to create their projects based on the acquired information. They created virtual public and private spaces populated by objects, stories, and discussion cases and engaged in both synchronous and asynchronous conversations. The activities in Zora encouraged students to work on personally meaningful issues. For example, some students chose to focus on the role of the universities, in particular the education, child development, and psychology departments, to provide child care and educational opportunities for members of the surrounding communities. The resulting virtual house was called *No Preschooler Left Behind*. It consisted of 77 virtual objects and was divided into two sections—the first was structured as a town hall for discussion, and the second was decorated as a preschool with play areas. In the No Preschooler Left Behind discussion town hall, there were 26 message boards, each with a thought-provoking question to spark discussion. A number of photographs also accompanied these message boards.
- *Creativity.* Students used different media in Zora to express different aspects of civic engagement. While creating online projects, students developed a sense of *confidence* in their creative potential. During the three-day ACT program students created their own virtual dorm rooms. They downloaded favorite sports team images, pictures of famous singers, and other images to decorate their virtual walls. In addition, the first cohort of ACT participants created 37 public spaces, such as the Mike Jones Student Center, the Sports Center, the Math and Science Building, the Orwell Language Hall, the Winifred Mandela Library, and a total of 338 objects inside these public spaces. The second cohort created 19 public spaces, such as the Community Theatre, Healthy Start, Healthy Life house, No Preschooler Left Behind, and Diversity House, and a total of 4,726 objects.

- *Collaboration.* Students work together to make a virtual campus of the future and to determine policies to organize life on the future campus and the relationship with the neighboring community. Online deliberation around the issues they cared about was encouraged among students, as well as face-to-face activities.
- *Communication.* ACT was aimed at scaffolding the formation of a peer network to provide the social and emotional support needed by many young people who leave home for the first time and need to *connect* with peers or with peer mentors. For cohort 1, the Zora Activity Log recorded 2,286 lines of chat over the three days; whereas there were 3,612 lines of chat from cohort 2. They discussed issues such as student life, policies/rules for graduation, the Internet, administration, and student services. The following is an excerpt of an online conversation in which students in cohort 1 discussed funding for students' clubs:

    PETER: Are we going to have fun student clubs? Do clubs have to give back to the community?
      MELANIE: If you are giving back to the community, should you get more money?
      ALAN: Should we fund the clubs?
      PETER: Every year, they give their proposal . . . then they decide . . . and get their permission.
      DAVID: If you are giving back to the community, you should get money. Why put money into clubs?
      PETER: If it lasts then that is good; but if you are new, you start-off with the minimum amount.

- *Community building.* Each year participants hosted an open house at the end of the semester where they showed videos they made about their virtual campus. They invited campus faculty, staff, and students to visit the *Campus of the Future* they created in Zora. Participants introduced the audience to their virtual creations and shared their ideas for building a stronger community within the campus as well as strengthening the relationship between campus and the surrounding neighborhoods. For example, some students chose to focus on the relationship between the local town police and the university police by interviewing police officials to better understand if and how the surrounding communities benefit from the campus police. Based on this information, they created a virtual exhibit hall called the Police Case Study. This house contained 23 objects and four message boards to trigger discussion. For example, they included a comparison of salaries between the university and public police forces. This discussion topic

was accompanied by statistics as well as graphics displaying the types of jobs and roles on each of the police forces.
- *Choices of conduct.* Youth engaged in the creation of a collaborative values dictionary to guide actions in the virtual world and by inhabiting the virtual campus of the future. For example, cohort 1 logged 36 values entries and 80 definitions in the values dictionary. Some of the values were *academic curiosity,* defined as "keeping your mind open to diversity in learning"; *integrity,* defined as "keeping to one's morals"; *tolerance,* defined as "the ability to not allow differences to get between you and others"; and *trust,* defined as "knowing that others will not take advantage of your vulnerabilities."

Next, I am presenting the PTD framework as it informs the concrete practice of the ACT program (see Figure 12.8).

DESIGN DIMENSIONS

Youth participation in the 2008 U.S. electoral campaign sparked interest and debates regarding youth engagement in civic and political activities.

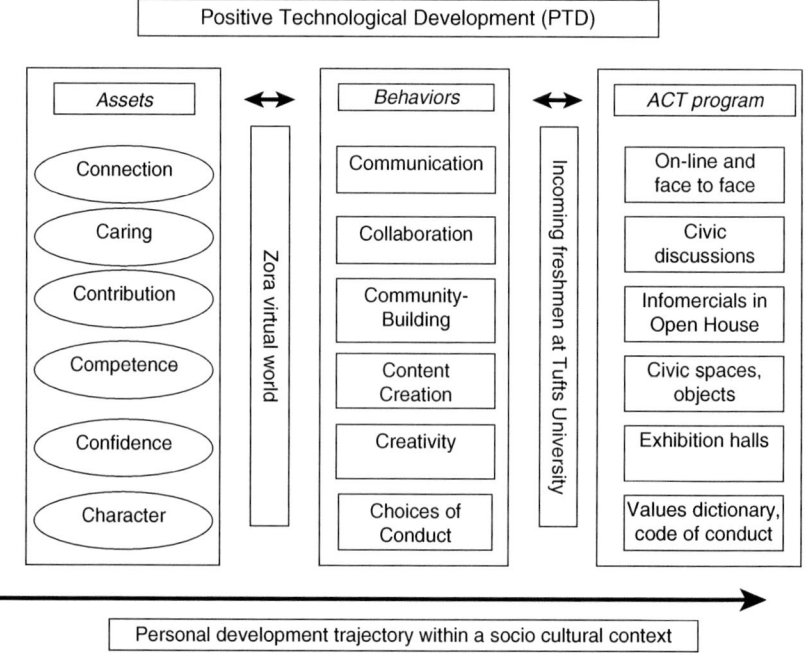

Figure 12.8. The PTD framework as it informs the ACT program.

According to the Center for Information and Research on Civic Learning and Engagement (2008), youth voter turnout was estimated between 52% and 53%, an increase of more than 10 percentage points over the last decade, and was comparable to the all-time highest turnout in 1972, when 18 year olds could first vote. It seems that often-cited criticisms of youth apathy or disengagement from public and civic activities might need to be revisited (Keeter et al., 2002; Michelsen, Zaff, & Hair, 2002). If voter turnout is an indicator, youth civic engagement has resurged since the steady decline that began three decades ago, a decline some researchers attributed to young people's loss of trust and confidence in institutionalized activities, especially those regarded as remote, opaque, and difficult to control (Grant Maker Forum on Community & National Service, 2001; Levine & Lopez, 2002).

This recent trend in youth engagement might be related to the emergence of new forms of youth civic activities that involve the use of new technologies (Bennett, 2007). The Internet can be a venue for helping young people to develop a sense of volunteerism and activism, for engaging in new forms of civic activities such as online petitioning and civic dialogues, and for promoting traditional types of civic activities such as voting (Williams, 2006a). Furthermore, virtual world programs can be explicitly designed to promote civic engagement (Bers, 2008c; Cassell, 2002). The Zora-based ACT program is an example.

1. Developmental Milestones

Youth in late adolescence, around 17 and 18 years old, are experiencing a period characterized by Erikson as *identity* vs. *role confusion*. The young person is struggling with the question, "Who am I, and where am I going?" as she is trying to achieve the developmental milestone of fidelity, or the ability to sustain loyalties in spite of contradictions in value systems. As they make the transition from childhood to adulthood, adolescents ponder the roles they will play in the adult world and the worldviews they will embrace. They are at a crossroads where decisions happen, in terms of both career choice and political orientation.

2. Curriculum

The ACT curriculum focuses on the theme of designing a *Campus of the Future* and is designed upon notions of social justice. It engages students in three types of experiences: (1) conducting research about campus, communities, and civic issues; (2) using Zora for discussion, collaborative design, and creation of virtual exhibits; and (3) creating a final ACT video to share with the university community. While the curriculum has specific topics for students to explore through discussion cases (e.g., youth programs, safety, equity, private/public funds), participants are able to create the Campus of the Future to reflect upon issues they are most interested in. The curriculum starts with open-ended suggested activities to help students get to know each other and the college campus and purposefully requires them to engage in deliberation and voting activities (see Table 12.5).

3. Technology

The ACT program uses the Zora virtual world as a platform for participants to create their virtual campus of the future and related exhibits.

Table 12.5. SAMPLE ACTIVITIES FROM THE ACT CURRICULUM

Activity	Goal	Description
Scavenger Hunt and Meet the Leaders	To give a chance for participants to learn about the community and speak to various leaders on campus and in the community to learn about vexing issues.	(1) Participants engage in a scavenger hunt to visit various important locations on campus and in the community; and (2) Participants meet campus administrators, student group leaders, and community officials to learn about their work in the community.
Designing the Details: Building the Campus of the Future	(1) To encourage participants to reflect on their research; and (2) To spark discussions about what they can do as students regarding the issues they learned about in the previous activity.	Participants collaboratively create various public exhibits to display their research and ideas regarding ways in which members of their Campus of the Future can engage in civic activities.
A Personality of Its Own: Giving Your Campus Values, Heroes, and Rules	To spark discussions about sources of positive and negative impact on campus and in the community.	(1) Participants create and share values and definitions in the collaborative values dictionary; (2) Participants create, as a group, a Campus Code of Ethics to summarize rules by which members of their Campus of the Future are bounded; and (3) Participants contribute objects about people and organizations that they think have positive and negative impacts on their community to a Gallery of Heroes and a Gallery of Villains.

Table 12.5. (CONTINUED)

Activity	Goal	Description
A Test of Strength: Dealing With Real-Life Campus Decisions	(1) To help participants critically think about the design of their Campus of the Future; and (2) To suggest new design ideas.	Participants read news article clippings regarding university decisions on topics related to civic engagement on campus. Participants are asked to reflect on these news items and are challenged to think about how and whether their Campus of the Future would handle similar issues.
Lights, Camera, Action! Creating Video Infomercials	(1) To encourage participants to think about the key aspects of their experience; and (2) To provide participants a means to conclude and archive their work and to showcase their experience during an open house event.	Participants create a short infomercial about their Campus of the Future; each student takes on a different role in the video production.

4. Mentoring Model

The ACT program was designed as a college pre-orientation program. Mentors were upperclassmen who received training. Besides providing technical support and guiding participants through the activities, peer leaders took part in designing the curriculum and activities outside of the computer labs. Including peer leaders in the design process was critical in fostering the mentoring relationship between the peer leaders and participants. The intention was to provide a genuine experience for both the peer leaders and the participants to build a mentoring relationship that could last beyond the three-day program. The success of the ACT mentoring model was evident in that over half of the first-year participants volunteered, without prompt, to return as peer leaders for the second year.

5. Diversity

The issue of diversity for this program rested in technical competency, previous experience with civic or community-related activities, and exposure to the community neighboring the university. ACT selected students with a range of technological experience and from different types of communities. Through our analysis of the Zora logs and field notes, we found patterns in Zora interactions that could be attributed to the diversity of participants' backgrounds. For example, participants who reported being less savvy with social media, including one participant who had a difficult time keeping up with typing in chat, tended to be more active building objects than engaging in online conversations.

6. Project Scale

ACT was designed as a pilot orientation program funded by a grant for a small number of participants. Only 18 participants and four peer mentors were accepted each year of the program. The small scale was purposefully designed to test whether the university could uptake the program and could scale it to offer for all students on campus.

7. Type of Contact With Participants

Unlike the other case studies described in this chapter and similar projects conducted by other researchers using virtual environments (Barab et al., 2005; Dede et al., 2005), the ACT program included approximately equal time for online and for face-to-face interaction. This was purposefully designed to reflect the overall goal of the program and the curriculum. The small group needed to form a peer network that could successfully work together collaboratively in a brief amount of time. The hope was that relationships formed could extend beyond the program. Thus face-to-face time was deemed equally important as online time. ACT was designed to maximize the relationship-building aspects of the program face-to-face (e.g., social activities, learning about the community and the campus environment) and the curricular aspects of building the Campus of the Future online. Over the three days, participants logged into Zora for ACT activities for approximately 26.5 hours and spent approximately 27 hours in noncomputer orientation activities such as taking the campus tour, orientation lectures, dining out, and social activities.

8. Assessment

The purpose of this study was to first understand the characteristics of students who chose to sign up for the ACT program, in particular to evaluate if there were individual characteristics, such as technological competency, and inclination toward civic participation that attracted students to this program versus other pre-orientation programs offered by the university. The second objective was to examine potential patterns in the way participants used Zora to promote and support discussions, activities, and research regarding civic engagement. Third, we examined participants' reactions and response to the ACT program. Last, we measured the carryover, longitudinal effect of the ACT program on participants' civic attitudes and engagement as compared with participants from other college orientation programs (Bers & Chau, 2006, 2010). Assessing participants' experience included multiple modes of data collection, such as Zora logs, and completion of the Positive Technological Development Questionnaire (Bers, 2006; Bers et al., 2009) before, after, and during a three-month follow-up to the program to assess attitude changes toward technologies, competencies, and experience as a result of the program. Results relating to these data are reported in Bers & Chau, 2010. In addition, participants were interviewed right after the program and six months later.

9. Access Environment

The ACT program was held at monitored and supported computer labs on campus. This added to the smooth operation of the various activities. While Zora could be installed on most student computers, the decision to administer the program at the labs was to ensure reliability and consistency and to secure support from the university IT staff. Although most curricular activities were conducted in the Zora virtual world, there were certain interactions that participants found to be more efficient, or more possible, via face-to-face discussion. Because participants only had a brief amount of time allocated for this program, they were rushed to gain fluency in the Zora interface and to design a virtual exhibit. Certain elements of the future campus that participants felt were less pertinent, such as the placement of specific virtual houses or signs, they decided to work out through face-to-face interactions.

10. Institutional Context of Usage

The ACT program was situated within the context of other established pre-orientations within the university such as fitness and outdoor exploration programs. ACT was the only one that focused on the relationship between the neighborhood community and the students as members of a university campus. The ACT program goals were aligned with a push from the university administration to promote civic engagement among the student body. As a program offered for university students, and because it was held in a monitored space, the program received adequate IT support. In terms of discipline, the program adhered to university rules; however, not enough thought was put into discussing how these rules would translate into the virtual world to address disciplinary issues.

Conclusion

This book presents new ideas for understanding the role of the digital landscape in youth development. While much has been written about the uses and abuses of new technologies by children and teenagers, there is very little to help us make sense not only of the vast opportunities that these new spaces offer for development but of general principles for designing these spaces. By introducing spatial metaphors, such as "playpens vs. playgrounds," "parks vs. malls," and "wireless hangouts vs. palaces in time," I hope to bring forward the essential developmental tasks that children face as they grow from toddlers to adolescents. It is not about the spaces per se but about the kinds of experiences these spaces support. The same is true with new technologies. Regardless of the bells and whistles, not all technologies can be used in open-ended ways to promote positive youth development. In this book I advocate for digital landscapes that engage children in playful learning by supporting content creation, creativity, choices of conduct, communication, collaboration, and community building. These are the six C's proposed by the Positive Technological Development framework. They can guide the design and the evaluation of experiences from early childhood to adolescence.

Over almost the last two decades I have done applied research in this area, and I have spent years working with children and the adults in their lives—parents, teachers, and doctors. I have designed and evaluated robotic platforms, virtual worlds, programming languages, and storytelling systems for children. Based on all of this experience, I developed Positive Technological Development, a framework for conceiving programs that make use of new technologies to promote positive youth development. The PTD framework invites readers to see themselves as co-designers of the digital landscape by focusing on positive behaviors that can be promoted by new technologies.

I conceive new technologies as spaces where development happens, as opposed to instruments to achieve certain goals. Thus, like any other spaces, new technologies can be designed to promote or hinder development.

This book hopes to shift the public discussion from a deficit paradigm to a positive and asset-promotion discourse. The digital landscape is here to stay. It is our role as adults to understand how we can become its co-designers so that children can have the best possible experiences with technology. Although the book presents a hopeful account for designing digital landscapes to promote positive youth development, it also offers a cautionary note about the dangers of taking a "technocentric approach" and assuming that new technologies are more powerful in their impact than the social, cultural, and economical structures that are currently in place.

Researchers in the social sciences have used descriptive approaches for understanding children and technology. Since Sherry Turkle's pioneer work published in *The Second Self* (1984) and her most recent work in *Alone Together* (2010), researchers have recognized the importance of technology in children's lives and have observed and analyzed how young people use, appropriate, and assign meaning to the technologies around them. Turkle's early work focused on the first generation of children who played with "smart" toys. Her research aimed at understanding how those electronic toys elicited thinking about self and identity. As one of my mentors at MIT, Sherry Turkle taught me the importance of computational objects as psychological tools that provide windows into children's development. In this book, I extend the metaphor from tools to spaces, as the new technologies of this decade are as much about social interactions as about industriousness.

But I also depart from the social sciences in my interventionist approach. I am a designer at heart. I did my doctoral work at the MIT Media Lab, where people invent the future, as opposed to describe it. Although I want to understand, I want even more to make things happen. My goal with this book is to provide intellectual tools for those who develop psychoeducational programs and innovative digital landscapes for youth learning and development. This work is interdisciplinary, but it is guided by a designer's mentality: not design for the sake of usability, or design for the sake of aesthetics, but design for the sake of positive youth development.

This book is also about values. It is about leveraging the potential of new technologies to support personal development and social change. It is about a commitment to make a better world with the tools that we have available in the 21st century. But it is also a vision for maintaining what is unique about being human, even when the tools of the next century might be different from those we know today.

This book is for people who are interested in learning how today's children are participating in the digital landscape. But it is also for people who want to have an impact. It is for those who want to craft educational and psychosocial programs in the technological space and for those who already have running programs but want to bring them into the 21st century by incorporating digital tools. And it is for parents who want to facilitate the best possible digital experiences for their children. This book is for all who might not love technology per se but who understand its potential for positive youth development. It is my hope that this book offers a possible path to help children out of the playpens and onto the playgrounds of this technological era.

References

Aries, P. (1960). *Centuries of childhood*. Harmondsworth, UK: Penguin Education.

Association of Virtual Worlds. (2008, August). *The blue book: A consumer guide to virtual worlds*. Retrieved February 10, 2009, from http://www.associationofvirtualworlds.com/publishing_blue_book.php

Aviram, R., & Eshet-Alkalai, Y. (2006). Towards a theory of digital literacy: Three scenarios for the next steps. *European Journal of Open Distance E-Learning*. Retrieved August 20, 2010, from http://www.eurodl.org/materials/contrib/2006/Aharon_Aviram.htm

Ba, H., Tally, W., & Tsikalas, K. (2002). Investigating children's emerging digital literacies. *Journal of Technology, Learning, and Assessment, 1*(4), 1–48.

Barab, S., & Squire, K. (2004). Design-based research: Putting a stake in the ground. *Journal of the Learning Sciences, 13*(1), 1–14.

Barab, S. A., Thomas, M., Dodge, T., Carteaux, R., & Tuzun, H. (2005). Making learning fun: Quest Atlantis, a game without guns. *Educational Technology Research and Development, 53*(1), 86–108.

Barron, B. (2004). Learning ecologies for technological fluency: Gender and experience differences. *Journal of Educational Computing Research, 31*(1), 1–36.

Bateson, G. (1972). *Steps to an ecology of mind: Collected essays in anthropology, psychiatry, evolution, and epistemology*. Chicago: University of Chicago Press.

Beals, L. (2011). *A framework for the design and evaluation of virtual world programs for preadolescent youth* (Unpublished doctoral dissertation). Tufts University, Medford, MA.

Beals, L., & Bers, M. U. (2009). A developmental lens for designing virtual worlds for children and youth. *International Journal of Learning and Media, 1*(1), 51–65.

Beals, L., & Bers, M. U. (2010). Evaluating participation in an international bilingual virtual world educational intervention for youth. *Journal of Virtual Worlds Research, 2*(5). Retrieved from http://ase.tufts.edu/Devtech/publications/metaverse.pdf

Bennett, W. L. (Ed.). (2007). *Civic life online. Learning how digital media can engage youth*. Cambridge, MA: MIT Press.

Benson, P. L., Scales, P. C., Hamilton, S. F., & Sesma, A., Jr. (2006). Positive youth development: Theory, research, and applications. In R. M. Lerner (Ed.), *Theoretical models of human development*, vol. 1 of *Handbook of child psychology* (6th ed.). Hoboken, NJ: Wiley.

Berk, L. E. (2008). *Exploring lifespan development*. Boston, MA: Allyn & Bacon.

Bers, M. (1998). A constructionist approach to values through on-line narrative tools. In *Proceedings of International Conference for the Learning Sciences (ICLS'98)*, (pp. 49–55). Chicago: AACE.

Bers, M. (1999). Narrative construction kits: Who am I? Who are you? What are we? In *Proceedings of Narrative Intelligence Fall Symposium*, AAAI'99 (pp. 44–51).

Bers, M. (2001). Identity construction environments: Developing personal and moral values through the design of a virtual city. *Journal of the Learning Sciences, 10*(4), 365–415.

Bers, M. (2003a). We are what we tell: Designing narrative environments for children. In P. Sengers & M. Mateas (Eds.), *Narrative intelligence* (pp. 44–51). Amsterdam: John Benjamins.

Bers, M. (2003b). Kaleidostories: Teachers and students creating a cross cultural virtual community through narrative. *Convergence: The Journal of Research Into New Media Technologies, 9*(2), 54–58.

Bers, M. (2006). The role of new technologies to foster positive youth development. *Applied Developmental Science, 10*(4), 200–219.

Bers, M. (2007a). Project InterActions: A multigenerational robotic learning environment. *Journal of Science and Technology Education, 16*(6), 537–552.

Bers, M. (2007b). Positive Technological Development: Working with computers, children, and the Internet. *MassPsych, 51*(1), 5–7, 18–19.

Bers, M. (2008a). *Blocks to robots: Learning with technology in the early childhood classroom.* New York: Teachers College Press.

Bers, M. (2008b). Engineers and storytellers: Using robotic manipulatives to develop technological fluency in early childhood. In O. Saracho & B. Spodek (Eds.), *Contemporary perspectives on science and technology in early childhood education* (pp. 105–125). Charlotte, NC: Information Age Publishing.

Bers, M. (2008c). Civic identities, online technologies: From designing civic curriculum to supporting civic experiences. In W. L. Bennett (Ed.), *Civic life online: Learning how digital media can engage youth* (pp. 139–160). (John D. and Catherine T. MacArthur Foundations Series on Digital Media and Learning). Cambridge, MA: MIT Press.

Bers, M. (2008d). A palace in time: Supporting children's spiritual development through new technologies. In R. Lerner, R. Roeser, & E. Phelps (Eds.), *Youth, development and spirituality: From theory to research* (pp. 339–358). West Conshohocken, PA: Templeton Foundation Press.

Bers, M. (2008e). Virtual worlds as digital playgrounds. *EDUCAUSE Review, 43*(5), 80–81.

Bers, M. (2009). New media for new organs: A virtual community for pediatric post-transplant patients. *Convergence: The Journal of Research Into New Media Technologies, 15*(4), 462–469.

Bers, M. (2010a). When robots tell a story about culture . . . and children tell a story about learning. In N. Yelland (Ed.), *Contemporary perspective on early childhood education* (pp. 227–247). Maidenhead, UK: Open University Press.

Bers, M. (2010b). The TangibleK Robotics Program: Applied computational thinking for young children. *Early Childhood Research and Practice, 12*(2). Retrieved from http://ecrp.uiuc.edu/v12n2/bers.html

Bers, M. (2010c). Let the games begin: Civic playing on high-tech consoles. *Review of General Psychology, 14*(2), 147–153.

Bers, M. (2010d). Beyond computer literacy: Supporting youth's positive development through technology. *New Directions for Youth Development, 128*, 13–23.

Bers, M. (2010e, Winter). New directions for youth development. Special issue, *New Media and Technology: Youth as Content Creators, 128*.

Bers, M., Ackermann, E., Cassell, J., Donegan, B., Gonzalez-Heydrich, J., DeMaso, D., et al. (1998). Interactive storytelling environments: Coping with cardiac illness at Boston's Children's Hospital. In *Proceedings of Computer–Human Interaction (CHI'98)* (pp. 603–609). Los Angeles: ACM.

Bers, M., Beals, L., Chau, C., Satoh, K., Blume, B., DeMaso, D., & Gonzalez-Heydrich, J. (2010). Use of a virtual community as a psychosocial support system in pediatric transplantation [Editorial]. *Pediatric Transplantation, 14*, 261–267.

Bers, M., Beals, L., Chau, C., Satoh, K., & Khan, N. (2010). Virtual worlds for young people in a program context: Lessons from four case studies. In M. Khine & I. Saleh (Eds.), *New science of learning: Cognition, computers, and collaboration in education* (pp. 357–383). New York: Springer Publishing Co.

Bers, M., & Cassell, J. (1998). Interactive storytelling systems for children: Using technology to explore language and identity. *Journal of Interactive Learning Research, 9*(2), 183–215.

Bers, M., & Chau, C. (2006). Fostering civic engagement by building a virtual city. *Journal of Computer-Mediated Communication, 11*(3). Retrieved from http://jcmc.indiana.edu/vol11/issue3/bers.html

Bers, M., & Chau, C. (2010). The virtual campus of the future: Stimulating and simulating civic actions in a virtual world. *Journal of Computing in Higher Education, 22*(1), 1–23.

Bers, M., Chau, C., Satoh, K., & Beals, L. (2007). Virtual communities of care: Online peer networks with post-organ transplant youth. In *Proceedings of the 2007 Computer Supported Collaborative Learning Conference, New Brunswick, NJ*.

Bers, M., Gonzalez-Heydrich, J., & DeMaso, D. (2001). Identity construction environments: Supporting a virtual therapeutic community of pediatric patients undergoing dialysis. In *Proceedings of Computer–Human Interaction (CHI'01)* (pp. 380–387). Seattle: ACM.

Bers, M., Gonzalez-Heydrich, G., & DeMaso, D. (2002). Future of technology to augment patient support in hospitals. *Studies in Health, Technology and Informatics, 80*, 231–244.

Bers, M., Gonzalez-Heydrich, G., & DeMaso, D. (2003, April). Use of a computer-based application in a pediatric hemodialysis unit: A pilot study. *Journal of the American Academy of Child and Adolescent Psychiatry, 42*(4), 493–496.

Bers, M., Gonzalez-Heydrich, G., DeMaso, D., Corsini, E., & Harmon, W. (2000, May). *Zora: A pilot virtual community in the pediatric dialysis unit* [Abstract]. American Society for Pediatrics Meeting, Boston, MA.

Bers, M., Gonzalez-Heydrich, J., Raches, D., & DeMaso, D. (2001). *Zora: A pilot virtual community in the pediatric dialysis unit*. Amsterdam: IOS Press.

Bers, M., & Horn, M. (2010). Tangible programming in early childhood: Revisiting developmental assumptions through new technologies. In I. R. Berson & M. J. Berson (Eds.), *High-tech tots: Childhood in a digital world* (pp. 49–70). Greenwich, CT: Information Age Publishing.

Bers, M., Lynch, A. D., & Chau, C. (Forthcoming). Positive technological development: The multifaceted nature of youth technology use towards improving self and society. In C. C. Ching & B. J. Foley (Eds.), *Technology, learning, and identity: Research on the development and exploration of selves in a digital world*. Cambridge: Cambridge University Press.

Bers, M., New, B., & Boudreau, L. (2004). Teaching and learning when no one is expert: Children and parents explore technology. *Journal of Early Childhood Research and Practice*. Retrieved from http://ase.tufts.edu/devtech/publications/teaching-learning.pdf

Bers, M., Ponte, I., Juelich, K., Viera, A., & Schenker, J. (2002). Teachers as designers: Integrating robotics in early childhood education. *Information Technology in Childhood Education, Annual 2002 (1) AACE*, 123–145.

Bers, M., & Portsmore, M. (2005). Teaching partnerships: Early childhood and engineering students teaching math and science through robotics. *Journal of Science Education and Technology, 14*(1), 59–74.

Bers, M., & Urrea, C. (2000). Technological prayers: Parents and children exploring robotics and values. In A. Druin & J. Hendler (Eds.), *Robots for kids: Exploring new technologies for learning experiences* (pp. 194–217). New York: Morgan Kaufman.

Biermann, F., & Pattberg, P. (2008). Global environmental governance: Taking stock, moving forward. *Annual Review of Environment and Resources, 33*, 277–294.

Black, R. (2008). *Adolescents and online fan fiction*. New York: Peter Lang.

Blair, C. (2002). School readiness: Integrating cognition and emotion in a neurobiological conceptualization of children's functioning at school entry. *American Psychologist, 57*(2), 111–127.

Blatt, M., & Kohlberg, L. (1975). The effect of classroom moral discussion upon children's level of moral judgment. *Journal of Moral Education, 4*, 129–161.

Blumler, J. G., & Coleman, S. (2001). *Realising democracy online: A civic commons in cyberspace.* London: Institute or Public Policy Research/Citizens Online.

Brem, A., Brem, F., McGrath, M., & Spirito, A. (1988). Psychosocial characteristics and coping skills in children maintained on chronic dialysis. *Pediatric Nephrology, 2*(4), 460–465.

Brennan, K., Monroy-Hernandez, A., & Resnick, M. (2010). Making projects, making friends: Online community as catalyst for interactive media creation. *New Directions for Youth Development, 2010*(128), 75–83.

Bronson, P., & Merryman, A. (2010, July 10). The creativity crisis. *Newsweek.*

Brosterman, N. (1997). *Inventing kindergarten.* New York: H. N. Abrams.

Brown, T. (2009). *Change by design: How design thinking transforms organizations and inspires innovation.* New York: HarperCollins.

Bruckman, A. (1996). MOOSE Crossing: Creating a learning culture. In *Proceedings of the 1996 International Conference on Learning Sciences* (pp. 571–572). Evanston, IL: International Society of the Learning Sciences.

Bruckman, A. (1998). Community support for constructionist learning. *Computer Supported Cooperative Work, 7*(1–2), 47–86.

Buckingham, D. (2003). *Media education: Literacy, learning, and contemporary culture.* Cambridge: Polity Press.

Buckingham, D., & Willett, R. (2006). *Digital generations: Children, young people, and new media.* Mahwah, NJ: Lawrence Erlbaum Associates.

Calvert, S. (2002). Identity construction on the Internet. In S. Calvert, R. R. Cocking, & A. B. Jordan (Eds.), *Children in the Digital Age: Influences of electronic media on development* (pp. 57–70). Westport, CT: Greenwood Publishing Group.

Calvino, I. (1972). *Invisible cities.* Turin: Giulio Enaudi.

Cantrell, K., & Bers, M. (2010). Zora Camp4All: A virtual community to augment the hopefulness of pediatric camping. *Child Life Focus, 28*(3), 1–7.

Cantrell, K., Fischer, A., Bouzaher, A., & Bers, M. (2010). E-mentorship in virtual communities for youth transplant recipients. *Journal of Pediatric Oncology Nursing, 27*(6), 344–355.

Cassell, J. (2002). "We have these rules inside": The effects of exercising voice in a children's online forum. In S. Calvert, R. Cocking, & A. Jordan (Eds.), *Children in the Digital Age* (pp. 123–144). New York: Praeger Press.

Cassell, J., Huffaker, D., Tversky, D., & Ferriman, K. (2006). The language of online leadership: Gender, age and youth engagement on the Internet. *Developmental Psychology, 42*(3), 436–449.

Cassidy, S., & Eachus, P. (2002). Developing the Computer User Self-Efficacy (CUSE) scale: Investigating the relationship between computer self-efficacy, gender and experience with computers. *Journal of Educational Computing Research, 26*(2), 169–189.

Cejka, E., Rogers, C., & Portsmore, M. (2006). Kindergarten robotics: Using robotics to motivate math, science, and engineering literacy in elementary school. *International Journal of Engineering Education, 22*(4), 711–722.

Center for Information and Research on Civic Learning and Engagement. (2008). Retrieved from http://www.civicyouth.org/special-report-by-circle-and-rock-the-vote-young-voter-registration-and-turnout-trends/

Clements, D. H., & Sarama, J. (2003). Young children and technology: What does the research say? *Young Children, 58*(6), 34–40.

Coffin, R., & MacIntyre, P. D. (1999). Motivational influences on computer-related affective states. *Computers in Human Behavior, 15*, 549–569.

Coiro, J. (2003). Rethinking comprehension strategies to better prepare students for critically evaluating content on the Internet. *NERA Journal, 39*, 29–34.

Coiro, J., Knobel, M., Lankshear, C., & Leu, D. (Eds.). (2008). *The handbook of research on new literacies.* Mahwah, NJ: Erlbaum.

Colby, A., & Damon, W. (1992). *Some do care: Contemporary lives of moral commitment.* New York: Free Press.

Committee on Information Technology Literacy. (1999). *Being fluent with information technology.* Computer Science and Telecommunication Board, Commission on Physical Sciences, Mathematics, and Applications, National Research Council. Washington, DC: National Academy Press.

Cordes, C., & Miller, E. (2000). *Fool's gold: A critical look at computers in childhood.* College Park, MD: Alliance for Childhood. Retrieved June 17, 2004, from http://www.alliance forchildhood.net/projects/computers

Csikszentmihalyi, M. (2000). *Flow: The psychology of optimal experience.* New York: HarperCollins.

Csikszentmihalyi, M., & Rochberg-Halton, E. (1981). *The meaning of things domestic symbols and self.* Cambridge: Cambridge University Press.

Cunha, F., & Heckman, J. J. (2006). *Investing in our young people.* Alexandria, VA: America's Promise Alliance.

Damon, W. (1990). *The moral child: Nurturing children's natural moral growth.* New York: Free Press.

Damon, W. (2004). What is positive youth development? *Annals of the American Academy of Political and Social Science, 591*(1), 13–24.

Damon, W., Menon, J., & Bronk, C. K. (2003). The development of purpose during adolescence. *Applied Developmental Sciences, 7*, 119–128.

Dede, C., Ketelhut, D. J., Clarke, J., Nelson, B., & Bowman, C. (2005). *Students' motivation and learning of science in a multi-user virtual environment.* Paper presented at the American Educational Research Association Conference, Montreal, Canada.

Dede, C., Nelson, B., Ketelhut, D. J., Clarke, J., & Bowman, C. (2004). Design-based research strategies for studying situated learning in a multi-user virtual environment. In *Proceedings of the 6th International Conference on Learning Sciences* (pp. 158–165). Santa Monica, CA: International Society of the Learning Sciences.

Druin, A. (2002). The role of children in the design of new technology. *Behavior and Information Technology, 21*(1), 1–25.

Earl, J., & Schussman, A. (2008). Contesting cultural control: Youth culture and online petitioning. In W. L. Bennett (Ed.), *Civic life online: Learning how digital media can engage youth* (pp. 71–96). (John D. and Catherine T. MacArthur Foundation Series on Digital Media and Learning). Cambridge: MIT Press.

Edwards, B. (2007). *The history of Civilization.* Retrieved from http://www.gamasutra.com/view/feature/1523/the_history_of_civilization.php

Engle, D. (2001). Psychosocial aspects of the organ transplant experience: What has been established and what we need for the future. *Journal of Clinical Psychology, 57*, 521–549.

Entertainment Software Association. (2010). *Essential facts about the computer and the video game industry.* Retrieved February 28, 2011, from http://www.theesa.com/facts/pdfs/ESA_Essential_Facts_2010.PDF

Erikson, E. (1950). *Childhood and society.* New York: W. W. Norton.

Erikson, E. (1963). *Childhood and society* (2nd ed.). New York: Norton.

Erikson, E. (1982). *The life cycle completed: A review.* New York: Norton.

Erikson, E. (2000). Insight and responsibility (1964). In R. Coles (Ed.), *The Erik Erikson reader*. New York: W. W. Norton.
Eshet-Alkalai, Y. (2004). Digital literacy: A conceptual framework for survival skills in the digital era. *Journal of Multimedia and Hypermedia, 13*(1), 93–106.
Eshet-Alkalai, Y., & Chajut, E. (2009). Changes over time in digital literacy. *CyberPsychology and Behavior*. doi: 10.1089/cpb.2008.0264.
Ford, A. (1994). *Navegaciones: Comunicación, cultura y crisis*. Buenos Aires: Amorrurtu.
Gee, J. P. (2003). *What video games have to teach us about learning*. New York: Palgrave.
Gee, J. P. (2007). *Good video games + good learning*. New York: Peter Lang.
Gerson, A. C., Furth, S. L., Neu, A. M., & Fivush, B. A. (2004). Assessing associations between medication adherence and potentially modifiable psychosocial variables in pediatric kidney transplant recipients and their families. *Pediatric Transplantation, 8*, 543–550.
Gilligan, C. (1982). *In a different voice*. Cambridge, MA: Harvard University Press.
Grant Maker Forum on Community & National Service. (2001). *From inspiration to participation. A review of perspectives on youth civic engagement*. Report. Berkeley: Philanthropy for Active Civic Engagement.
Griffin, K. J., & Elkin, T. D. (2001). Non-adherence in pediatric transplantation: A review of the existing literature. *Pediatric Transplantation, 5*(4), 246–249.
Grudin, J. (1994). Computer-supported cooperative work: History and focus. *Computer, 27*(5), 19–26.
Grüsser, S. M., Thalemann, R., & Griffiths, M. (2007). Excessive computer game playing: Evidence for addiction and aggression? *CyberPsychology and Behavior, 10*, 290–292.
Heckman, J. J., & Masterov, D. V. (2004). *The productivity argument for investing in young children*. (Working Paper 5). Chicago: Invest in Kids Working Group, Committee for Economic Development.
Herring, S. (2002). Computer-mediated communication on the Internet. *Annual Review of Information Science and Technology, 36*(1), 109–168.
Heschel, A. J. (1951). *The Sabbath: It's meaning for modern man*. New York: Noonday.
Hoffman, M., & Blake, J. (2003). Computer literacy: Today and tomorrow. *Journal of Computing Sciences in Colleges, 18*(5), 221–233.
Horn, M. S., Bers, M. U., & Jacob, R. J. K. (2009, April). *Tangible programming in education: A research approach*. Paper presented at CHI '09, Boston, MA.
Horn, M. S., Crouser, R. J., & Bers, M. U. (2011). Tangible interaction and learning: The case for a hybrid approach. Special issue on tangibles and children, *Personal and Ubiquitous Computing*. doi: 10.1007/s00779-011-0404-2.
Horn, M. S., & Jacob, R. J. K. (2007). Designing tangible programming languages for classroom use. In B. Ullmer, A. Schmidt, E. Hornecker, C. Hummels, R. J. K. Jacob, & E. van den Hoven, *TEI '07: Proceedings of the First International Conference on Tangible and Embedded Interaction* (pp. 159–162). New York: Association for Computing Machinery.
Ito, M., Horst, H. A., Bittanti, M., boyd, D., Herr-Stephenson, B., Lange, P., et al. (2009). *Living and learning with new media: Summary of findings from the Digital Youth Project*. (John D. and Catherine T. MacArthur Foundation Reports on Digital Media Learning). Cambridge, MA: MIT Press.
James, C., Davis, K., Flores, A., Francis J., Pettingill, L., Rundle, M., & Gardner, H. (2009). *Young people, ethics, and the new digital media: A synthesis from the Good Play Project*. Cambridge, MA: MIT Press.
Jenkins, H. (2006). *Convergence culture: Where old and new media collide*. New York: New York University Press.
Jenkins, H. (2009). *Confronting the challenges of participatory culture: Media education for the 21st century*. Cambridge, MA: MIT Press.

Jenkins, H., Purushotma, R., Clinton, K., Weigel, M., & Robison, A. (2006). *Confronting the challenges of participatory culture: Media education for the 21st century*. Chicago, IL: MacArthur Foundation.

Josephson Institute of Ethics. (2008). *Character study reveals predictors of lying and cheating*. Retrieved February 28, 2011, from http://josephsoninstitute.org/surveys/index.html

Kafai, Y. B., & Resnick, M. (1996). *Constructionism in practice: Designing, thinking, and learning in a digital world*. Mahwah, NJ: Erlbaum.

Kahne, J., Middaugh, E., & Evans, C. (2008). *The civic potential of video games*. (MacArthur Foundation White Paper). Chicago: John D. and Catherine T. MacArthur Foundation.

Kaiser Report. (2010). *Generation M2: Media in the lives of 8- to 18-year olds*. Menlo Park, CA: Henry J. Kaiser Family Foundation.

Kantor, R., Elgas, P. M., & Fernie, D. E. (1989). First the look and then the sound: Creating conversations at circle time. *Early Childhood Research Quarterly, 4*(4), 433–448.

Karlström, P., Cerratto-Pargman, T., & Knutsson, O. (2008). Literate tools or tools for literacy? *Digital Kompetanse. Nordic Journal of Digital Literacy, 3*(2), 97–112.

Kato, P. M., Cole, S. W., Bradlyn, A. S., & Pollock, B. H. (2008). A video game improves behavioral outcomes in adolescents and young adults with cancer: A randomized trial. *Pediatrics, 122*, e305–e317.

Kay, A. (2003). Interview with Alan Kay. *Computers in Entertainment, 1*(1), 8.

Kazakoff, E. R., & Bers, M. U. (2011, April 8–12). *The impact of computer programming on sequencing ability in early childhood*. Paper presented at the American Educational Research Association Conference, New Orleans.

Keeter, S., Zukin, C., Andolina, M., & Jenkins, K. (2002). *The civic and political health of the nation: A generational portrait*. College Park, MD: University of Maryland, Center for Information and Research on Civic Learning and Engagement.

King, P. E., & Furrow, J. L. (2004). Religion as a resource for positive youth development: Religion, social capital, and moral outcomes. *Developmental Psychology, 40*, 703–714.

Kist, W. (2007). Basement new literacies: Dialogue with a first-year teacher. *English Journal, 97*(1), 43–48.

Kohlberg, L. (1976). Moral stages and moralization: The cognitive-developmental approach. In T. Lickona (Ed.), *Moral development and behavior: Theory, research and social issues*. New York: Holt, Rinehart & Winston.

Kohlberg, L. (1985). The just community approach to moral education in theory and in practice. In M. Berkowitz & F. Oser (Eds.), *Moral education: Theory and application* (pp. 22–87). Hillsdale, NJ: Lawrence Erlbaum Associates.

Kolodner, J., Crismond, C., Gray, J., Holbrook, J., & Puntamhekar, S. (1998). Learning by design from theory to practice. In *Proceedings of the International Conference of the Learning Sciences* (pp. 16–22). Charlottesville, VA: Association for the Advancement of Computing in Education.

Koschmann, T. (1996). Paradigm shifts and instructional technology: An introduction. In T. Koschmann (Ed.), *CSCL: Theory and practice of an emerging paradigm* (pp. 1–23). Mahwah, NJ: Erlbaum.

Kraut, R., Kiesler, S., Boneva, B., Cummings, J., Helgeson, V., & Crawford, A. (2002). Internet paradox revisited. *Journal of Social Issues, 58*, 49–74.

KZero Research. (2008). *Virtual worlds total registered accounts*. Retrieved from http://www.kzero.co.uk/blog/wp-content/uploads/2008/05/virtual-world-numbers-q2-2008.jpg

Lankshear, C., & Knobel, M. (2006). *New literacies: Everyday practices and classroom learning* (2nd ed.). New York: Open University Press and McGraw-Hill.

Larson, R. W. (2000). Toward a psychology of positive youth development. *American Psychologist, 55*(1), 170–183.

Lave, J., & Wenger, E. (1991). *Situated learning. Legitimate peripheral participation.* Cambridge, UK: Cambridge University Press.

Lenhart, A., Kahne, J., Middaugh, E., MacGill, A., Evans, C., & Vitak, J. (2008). *Teens, video games, and civics.* Washington, DC: Pew Internet & American Life Project.

Lenhart, A., Purcell, K., Smith, A., & Zickuhr, K. (2010). *Social media and young adults.* Washington, DC: Pew Internet & American Life Project.

Lerner, R. (2002). *Concepts and theories of human development.* Hillsdale, NJ: Lawrence Erlbaum Associates.

Lerner, R. (2007). *The good teen.* New York: Three Rivers Press.

Lerner, R. M., Almerigi, J. B., Theokas, C., & Lerner, J. V. (2005). Positive youth development: A view of the issues. *Journal of Early Adolescence, 25*(1), 10–16.

Lerner, R. M., & Barton, C. E. (2000). Adolescents as agents in the promotion of their positive development: The role of youth actions in effective programs. In W. J. Perrig & A. Grob (Eds.), *Control of human behavior, mental processes, and consciousness: Essays in honor of the 60th birthday of August Flammer* (pp. 457–475). Mahwah, NJ: Erlbaum.

Lerner, R., Wertlieb, D., & Jacobs, F. (2003). Historical and theoretical bases of applied developmental science. In R. M. Lerner, D. Wertlieb, & F. Jacobs (Eds.), *Handbook of applied developmental science, vol. 1: Applying developmental science for youth and families: Historical and theoretical foundations* (pp. 1–28). Thousand Oaks, CA: Sage.

Leu, D. J. (2001). Exploring literacy on the Internet: Internet project: Preparing students for new literacies in a global village. *Reading Teacher, 54*(6), 568–572.

Leu, D. J., Kinzer, C. K., Coiro, J. L., & Cammack, D. W. (2004). Toward a theory of new literacies emerging from the Internet and other information and communication technologies. In R. B. Ruddell & N. J. Unrau (Eds.), *Theoretical models and processes of reading* (5th ed.; p. 1570). Newark, DE: International Reading Association.

Levine, P., & Lopez, M. (2002). *Youth voter turnout has declined by any measure.* Retrieved from Center for Information and Research on Civic Learning and Engagement, http://www.civicyouth.org/research/products/fact_sheets_outside.htm

Libman, N. (2011). *Exploring Jewish identity through robotics* (Unpublished master's thesis). Tufts University.

Lieberman, D. A. (2001). Management of chronic pediatric diseases with interactive health games: Theory and research findings. *Journal of Ambulatory Care Management, 24,* 26–38.

Livingstone, S. (2004). Media literacy and the challenge of new information and communication technologies. *Communication Review, 7*(1), 3–14.

Livingstone, S. (2009). *Children and the Internet: Great expectations, challenging realities.* Cambridge: Polity.

Luehrmann, A. (1981). Computer literacy: What should it be? *Mathematics Teacher, 74*(9), 682–686.

Luehrmann, A. (2002). Should the computer teach the student, or vice-versa? *Contemporary Issues in Technology and Teacher Education, 2*(3), 389–396.

Markus, M. L. (1987). Toward a "critical mass" theory of interactive media: Universal access, interdependence and diffusion. *Communications Research, 14,* 491–511.

Marsh, J., & Hallet, E. (Eds.). (2008). *Desirable literacies: Approaches to language and literacy in the early years* (2nd ed.). London: Sage.

Martin, F., Mikhak, B., Resnick, M., Silverman, B., & Berg, R. (2000). To mindstorms and beyond: Evolution of a construction kit for magical machines. In A. Druin & J. Hendler (Eds.), *Robots for kids: Exploring new technologies for learning* (pp. 9–33). San Francisco: Morgan Kaufmann.

McLuhan, M. (1964). *Understanding media.* New York: Mentor.

McMillan, D. W. (1996). Sense of community. *Journal of Community Psychology*, 24(4), 315–325.

McNerney, T. S. (2004). From turtles to tangible programming bricks: Explorations in physical language design. *Personal and Ubiquitous Computing*, 8(5), 326–337.

Michelsen, E., Zaff, J. F., & Hair, E. C. (2002). *Civic engagement programs and youth development: A synthesis*. Washington, DC: Child Trends.

Montgomery, K. (2008). Youth and digital democracy: Intersections of practice, policy, and the marketplace. In W. L. Bennett (Ed.), *Civic life online. Learning how digital media can engage youth* (pp. 25–49). (John D. and Catherine T. MacArthur Foundation Series on Digital Media and Learning). Cambridge, MA: MIT Press.

Montgomery, K., Gottlieb-Robles, B., & Larson, G. (2004). *Youth as e-citizens: Engaging the digital generation*. Washington, DC: Center for Social Media, School of Communication, American University.

Muller, A. A., & Perlmutter, M. (1985). Preschool children's problem-solving interactions at computers and jigsaw puzzles. *Journal of Applied Developmental Psychology*, 6, 173–186.

National Association for Media Literacy Education. (2009). *Core principles of media literacy education in the United States*. Detroit: National Association for Media Literacy Education.

New, R., & Cochran, M. (2007). *Early childhood education: An international encyclopedia* (vols. 1–4). Westport, CT: Praeger.

Oldenburg, R. (1997). *The great good place: Cafés, coffee shops, community centers, beauty parlors, general stores, bars, hangouts, and how they get you through the day*. New York: Marlowe.

Ondrejka, C. (2004). *Living on the edge: Digital worlds which embrace the real world*. (Linden Lab White Paper).

Oppenheimer, T. (2003). *The flickering mind: The false promise of technology in the classroom and how learning can be saved*. New York: Random House.

Papert, S. (1980). *Mindstorms: Children, computers, and powerful ideas*. New York: Basic Books.

Papert, S. (1987, January/February). Computer criticism vs. technocentric thinking. *Educational Researcher*, 16(1), 22–30.

Papert, S. (1993). *The children's machine: Rethinking school in the age of the computer*. New York: Basic Books.

Papert, S., & Harel, L. (1991). *Constructionism*. New York: Ablex.

Papert, S., & Resnick, M. (1995). *Technological fluency and the representation of knowledge*. (Proposal to the National Science Foundation). Cambridge, MA: MIT Media Laboratory.

Partnership for 21st Century Skills. (2007). Retrieved from http://www.p21.org/index.php?option=com_content&task=view&id=504&Itemid=185

Perkins, D. (1986). *Knowledge as design*. New York: Lawrence Erlbaum Associates.

Perlman, R. (1976). *Using computer technology to provide a creative learning environment for preschool children*. (AI Memo 360: Logo Memo No. 24). Cambridge, MA: MIT Artificial Intelligence Laboratory.

Piaget, J. (1962). *Play, dreams and imitation in childhood*. New York: Norton.

Piaget, J. (1965). *The child's conception of number*. New York: W. W. Norton & Co.

Piscitelli, A. (2002). *Ciberculturas 2.0. En la era de las máquinas inteligentes*. Buenos Aires: Paidos.

Preece, J. (2000). *Online communities: Designing usability, supporting sociability*. Chichester, UK: John Wiley & Sons.

Prensky, M. (2006). *Don't bother me mom: I'm learning*. St. Paul: Paragon House.

Prescott, L. (2007). *Virtual worlds ranking—Runescape #1: Hitscape*. Retrieved February 10, 2009, from http://weblogs.hitwise.com/leeannprescott/2007/04/virtual_worlds_ranking_runesca.html

Putnam, R. (2000). *Bowling alone: The collapse and revival of the American community*. New York: Simon & Schuster.
Raynes-Goldie, K., & Walker, L. (2008). Our space: Online civic engagement tools for youth. In W. L. Bennett (Ed.), *Civic life online. Learning how digital media can engage youth* (pp. 161–188). (John D. and Catherine T. MacArthur Foundation Series on Digital Media and Learning). Cambridge, MA: MIT Press.
Reed, D. (1997). *Following Kohlberg: Liberalism and the practice of democratic community*. Notre Dame, IN: University of Notre Dame Press.
Repenning, A., Webb, D., & Ioannidou, A. (2010). Scalable game design and the development of a checklist for getting computational thinking into public schools. In *SIGCSE 2010: Proceedings of the 41st ACM Technical Symposium on Computer Science Education*. New York: Association for Computing Machinery.
Resnick, M. (1994). *Turtles, termites, and traffic jams: Explorations in massively parallel microworlds*. Cambridge, MA: MIT Press.
Resnick, M. (2003, February). Playful learning and creative societies. *Education Update, 8*(6).
Resnick, M. (2006). Computer as paintbrush: Technology, play, and the creative society. In D. Singer, R. Golikoff, & K. Hirsh-Pasek (Eds.), *Play = learning: How play motivates and enhances children's cognitive and social-emotional growth*. Oxford: Oxford University Press.
Resnick, M. (2007a, June). *All I really need to know (about creative thinking) I learned (by studying how children learn) in kindergarten*. Paper presented at the ACM Creativity and Cognition Conference, Washington, DC.
Resnick, M. (2007b, December). Sowing the seeds for a more creative society. *Learning and Leading With Technology, 35*(4), 18–22.
Resnick, M., Berg, R., & Eisenberg, M. (2000). Beyond black boxes: Bringing transparency and aesthetics back to scientific investigation. *Journal of the Learning Sciences, 9*(1), 7–30.
Resnick, M., Bruckman, A., & Martin, F. (1996, September/October). Pianos not stereos: Creating computational construction kits. *Interactions, 3*(6), 41–50.
Resnick, M., Maloney, J., Monroy-Hernández, A., Rusk, N., Eastmond, E., Brennan, K., et al. (2009). Scratch: Programming for all. *Communications of the ACM, 52*(11), 60–67.
Resnick, M., Martin, F., Sargent, R., & Silverman, B. (1996). Programmable bricks: Toys to think with. *IBM Systems Journal, 35*(3–4), 443–452.
Rheingold, H. (2008). Using participatory media and public voice to encourage civic engagement. In W. L. Bennett (Ed.), *Civic life online. Learning how digital media can engage youth* (pp. 97–118). (John D. and Catherine T. MacArthur Foundation Series on Digital Media and Learning). Cambridge, MA: MIT Press.
Ribble, M., Bailey, G., & Ross, T. (2004). Digital citizenship: Addressing appropriate technology behavior. *Learning and Leading With Technology, 32*(1), 6–12.
Rinaldi, C. (1998). Projected curriculum constructed through documentation—"Progettazione." In C. Edwards, L. Gandini, & G. Forman (Eds.), *The hundred languages of children: The Reggio Emilia approach—advanced reflections* (2nd ed.; pp. 127–139). CT: Ablex Publishing Co.
Ritchie, R. (1995). *Primary design and technology: A process for learning*. London: David Fulton Publishers.
Rodin, G., & Voshart, K. (1987). Depressive symptoms and functional impairment in the medically ill. *General Hospital Psychiatry, 9*, 251–258.
Rogers, C., & Portsmore, M. (2001). Data acquisition in the dorm room: Teaching experimentation techniques using LEGO materials. In *The proceeds of the American Society of Engineering Education Annual Exposition and Conference, New Mexico, June 2001*.
Rogers, C., & Portsmore, M. (2004). Bringing engineering to elementary school. *Journal of STEM Education, 5*(3–4), 17–28.

Rubin, K. H., Bukowski, W., & Parker, J. (2006). Peer interactions, relationships, and groups. In N. Eisenberg (Ed.), *Handbook of child psychology: Social, emotional, and personality development* (6th ed.; pp. 571–645). New York: Wiley.

Rusk, N., Resnick, M., Berg, R., & Pezalla-Granlund, M. (2008). New pathways into robotics: Strategies for broadening participation. *Journal of Science Education and Technology, 17*(1), 59–69.

Satoh, K., McVey, M., Grogan, D., & Bers, M. (2006). Zora: Implementing Virtual Communities of Learning and Care (VCLC). Paper presented at the New Media Consortium Regional Conference, San Antonio, TX.

Sawyer, R. (2006a). *Explaining creativity: The science of human innovation.* New York: Oxford University Press.

Sawyer, R. (2006b). Educating for innovation. *Thinking Skills and Creativity, 1*(1), 41–48.

Scales, P., Benson, P. L., Leffert, N., & Blyth, D. A. (2000). Contribution of developmental assets to the prediction of thriving among adolescents. *Applied Developmental Science, 4*(1), 27–46.

Scales, P., Benson, P., & Mannes, M. (2006). The contribution to adolescent well-being made by nonfamily adults: An examination of developmental assets as contexts and processes. *Journal of Community Psychology, 34*(4), 401–413.

Selman, R. (2003). *The promotion of social awareness: Powerful lessons from the partnership of developmental theory and classroom practice.* New York: Russell Sage Foundation.

Shaffer, D. W. (2007). *How computer games help children learn.* New York: Palgrave Macmillan.

Sherrod, L., Flanagan, C., & Youniss, J. (2002). Dimensions of citizenship and opportunities for youth development: The what, why, when, where, and who of citizenship development. *Applied Developmental Science, 6*(4), 264–272.

Shore, R. (2008). *The power of pow! Wham! Children, digital media, and our nation's future: Three challenges for the coming decade.* New York: Joan Ganz Cooney Center at Sesame Workshop. Retrieved February 10, 2009, from http://www.joanganzcooneycenter.org/pdf/Challenge_Paper_ExecSummary.pdf

Smith, A. C. (2007). Using magnets in physical blocks that behave as programming objects. In B. Ullmer, A. Schmidt, E. Hornecker, C. Hummels, R. J. K. Jacob, & E. van den Hoven, *TEI '07: Proceedings of the First International Conference on Tangible and Embedded Interaction* (pp. 147–150). New York: Association for Computing Machinery.

Soloway, E. (1993). Should we teach students to program? *Communications of the ACM, 36*(10), 21–24.

Squire, K. (2011). *Video games and learning: Teaching and participatory culture in the digital age.* New York: Teachers College Press.

Squire, K., & Barab, S. (2004). Replaying history: Engaging urban underserved students in learning world history through computer simulation games. In *Proceedings of the International Conference of the Learning Sciences* (pp. 505–512). Santa Monica.

Squire, K., & the Games-to-Teach Research Team. (2003). Design principles of next-generation gaming for education. *Educational Technology, 43*(5), 17–23.

Steinkuehler, C. A. (2006). Where everybody knows your (screen) name: Online games as "third places." Paper presented at DiGRA 2005: Worlds in Play, Annual Conference of the Digital Games Research Association, Vancouver, Canada.

Stone, L. (1977). *The family, sex and marriage in England, 1500–1800.* New York: Harper & Row.

Subrahmanyam, K., & Greenfield, P. (2008). Online communication and adolescent relationship. *The Future of Children: Children and the Electronic Media, 18,* 118–146.

Subrahmanyam, K., Greenfield, P., Kraut, R., & Gross, E. (2001). The impact of computer use on children's and adolescents' development. *Journal of Applied Developmental Psychology, 22,* 7–30.

Suzuki, H., & Kato, H. (1995). Interaction-level support for collaborative learning: Algoblock—an open programming language. In J. L. Schnase & E. L. Cunnius (Eds.), *Proceedings of CSCL '95: The First International Conference on Computer Support for Collaborative Learning* (pp. 349–355). Mahwah, NJ: Erlbaum.

Theokas, C., & Lerner, R. M. (2006). Observed ecological assets in families, schools, neighborhoods: Conceptualization, measurement, and relations with positive and negative developmental outcomes. *Applied Development Science, 10*(2), 61–74.

Tiwari, N. (2007). *Webkinz: I fell in love with a cyber alley cat* [cited August 29, 2008]. Retrieved February 10, 2009, from http://www.news.com/Webkinz-I-fell-in-love-with-a-cyber-alley-cat/2100-1026_3-6182834.html

Turbak, F., & Berg, R. (2002). Robotic design studio: Exploring the big ideas of engineering in a liberal arts environment. *Journal of Science Education and Technology, 11*(3), 237–253.

Turkle, S. (1984). *The second self: Computers and the human spirit.* New York: Basic Books.

Turkle, S. (1995). *Life on the screen. Identity in the age of Internet.* New York: Simon & Schuster.

Turkle, S. (2010). *Alone together: Why we expect more from technology and less from each other.* New York: Basic Books.

Turkle, S., & Papert, S. (1992). Epistemological pluralism and the revaluation of the concrete. *Journal of Mathematical Behavior, 11*(1), 3–33.

Verba, S., Schlozman, K. L., & Brady, H. E. (1995). *Voice and equality: Civic voluntarism in American politics.* Cambridge, MA: Harvard University Press.

Vygotsky, L. S. (1978). *Mind in society: The development of higher psychological processes.* Cambridge, MA: Harvard University Press.

Wartella, E. A., & Jennings, N. (2000). Children and computers: New technology—old concerns. *The Future of Children: Children and Computer Technology, 10*(2), 31–43.

Wiener, N. (1948). *Cybernetics or control and communication in the animal and the machine.* New York: John Wiley & Sons.

Williams, D. (2006a). Why game studies now? Gamers don't bowl alone. *Games and Culture, 1*(1), 13–16.

Williams, D. (2006b). On and off the'Net: Scales for social capital in an online era. *Journal of Computer-Mediated Communication, 11*(2), 593–628.

Williamson, D. A. (2008). *Kids and teens: Virtual worlds open new universe.* Retrieved February 10, 2009, from http://www.emarketer.com/Report.aspx?code=emarketer_2000437&src=report_summary_reportsell

Wing, J. M. (2006). Computational thinking. *Communications of the ACM, 49*(3), 33–35. Retrieved June 10, 2010, from http://www.cs.cmu.edu/afs/cs/usr/wing/www/publications/Wing06.pdf

Wyeth, P., & Purchase, H. C. (2002). Tangible programming elements for young children. In L. Terveen (Ed.), *Changing the world, changing ourselves: CHI 2002, Minneapolis, Minn., U.S.A., 20–25 April, 2002: Extended abstracts* (pp. 774–775). New York: Association for Computing Machinery.

Youniss, J., McLellan, J., & Yates, M. (1997, March). What we know about engendering civic identity. *American Behavioral Scientist, 40*(5), 620–631.

INDEX

abstraction, 69
access environment, 138
   of ACT, 173
   of TangibleK program, 155
   of Zora virtual world, 165
ACS. *See* American Cancer Society
Active Citizenship Through Technology (ACT), 122, 165
   access environment of, 173
   assessment of, 172–73
   choice of conduct in, 168
   collaboration in, 167
   communication in, 167
   community building in, 167–68
   confidence in, 166
   connection in, 167
   contact with participants in, 172
   content creation in, 166
   context of institution in, 173–74
   creativity in, 166
   curriculum of, 169, 170*t*–171*t*
   design dimensions of, 168–74
   developmental milestones of, 169
   diversity of, 171–72
   mentoring model of, 171
   PTD framework and, 169*f*
   scale of, 172
   technology of, 170
   Zora virtual world with, 166–74
ActiveWorlds, 162
activism, 169
adolescence, 15
   behavior during, 16–17
   boundaries of, 53–54
   development and, 16–17, 46, 52
   identity *vs.* role confusion of, 52–53, 169
   online communication, 104
   self-reflection of, 55

social needs of, 52
text messaging and, 55
wireless hangouts of, 54–56
advertising, 36, 57
AgentSheets, 72–73
Alice programming language, 73
Alone Together (Turkle), 176
American Cancer Society (ACS), 123–24
analysis, 69
animation, 49
anime, 80, 97–98
applied developmental psychology, 6–7
Aries, Philippe, 16
art
   computers and, 48–49
   digital, 77–78
artificial intelligence, 7, 14
assessment, 138
   of ACT, 172–73
   of TangibleK program, 153–54
   of Zora virtual world, 164
assets. *See also specific types*
   interpersonal, 11
   intrapersonal, 11
   PTD, 10–12, 13*f*, 17–18
   PYD and, 15–18
Association of Virtual Worlds, 42–43
Atari, 96
authority, children's dependence on, 146
autonomy, 24, 25, 28
   playgrounds and, 22–23
   software for, 67
avatars, 25, 54, 93, 162

Barab, Sasha, 95, 121
Bateson, Gregory, 6

Beals, Laura, 33–35
behavior, 87
  adolescent, 16–17
  communication and, 102
  online, 99–100
  PTD, 11–12, 13f, 17–18
  video games and, 41
behaviorism, 7
Bell Laboratories, 101
Bers, Marina, 46–48, 135, 145
Bers, Tali, 89–90
BlizzCon, 60
Blocks to Robots: Learning With Technology in the Early Childhood Classroom (Bers, M.), 135, 145
blogging, 58, 60–61, 76, 113–15
boundaries, in adolescence, 53–54
Brennan, Karen, 48–49
Brown, Tim, 64

CAI. *See* computer-assisted instruction
Calvino, Italo, 45
Camp4All, 109–10
Cantrell, Kathryn A., 109–10
capitalism, 36
caring, 11, 12, 111, 142–43, 157
caring networks, 111
Cascading Style Sheets, 81
cause and effect, 24
channel, of communication, 101–2
character, 11, 12
character traits, 144, 158
chat, 103
Chau, Clement, 56–58
CHERP. *See* Creative Hybrid Environment for Robotic Programming
childhood
  early, 22
  history of, 16
children. *See also* adolescence
  communication of, 103
  computer projects of, 5–6
  computers for, 26–27, 30–31
  dependence on authority, 146
  design and, 64–65
  development of, 3–5
  evolution of adult perspective on, 16
  history of childhood, 16
  media use by, 40–41
  moral judgment of, 92
  self-expression of, 8
  space for, 3
  technological literacy of, 4, 5, 33
Children's Online Privacy Protection Act (COPPA), 133–34
choice of conduct, 12, 91, 97–100
  in ACT, 168
  in TangibleK program, 144–45, 155
  in Zora virtual world, 158
citizenship, 120, 122. *See also* Active Citizenship Through Technology
civic engagement, 42, 119–23, 169
civic identity, 131–32
Civilization, 42, 121
Club Penguin, 103
cognitivism, 7
collaboration, 12, 49, 112–13
  in ACT, 167
  definition of, 111
  in TangibleK program, 142, 143f, 155
  in Zora virtual world, 157
Committee on Information Technology Literacy, 9
communication, 12. *See also* wireless communication
  in ACT, 167
  of adolescents, online, 104
  behavior and, 102
  channel of, 101–2
  of children, 103
  computers and, 9, 105
  definition of, 101
  Internet, 102–3
  interpretation and, 102
  medium of, 102
  peer, 103
  playground approach to, 103
  playpen approach to, 103–4
  symbols and, 26
  in TangibleK program, 143–44, 155
  text messaging, 55
  transmission model of, 101–2
  wireless, 52
  in Zora virtual world, 157
community, 42
  games and, 59–60
  global, 60–61
  identity and, 53
  third places and formation of, 95
  transgender, 124–26
  value of, 48
  virtual, 54, 109–10

community building, 12, 119–21
  in ACT, 167–68
  in TangibleK program, 144, 155
  in Zora virtual world, 157–58
competence, 11–12, 74
  computational thinking, 68–69
  confidence and, 84
  content creation and increase of, 67–68, 141
  development of, 36–37
  Zora virtual world and, 156
computational thinking, 68–69
computer-assisted instruction (CAI), 7
computers. *See also* programming
  art and, 48–49
  for children, 26–27, 30–31
  communication and, 9, 105
  creativity and, 83
  games, 23, 35, 59–60
  interfaces, human, 65
  iPad, 30–31
  as learning tools, 14
  literacy, 8, 9, 39
  personal, 14
  play and, 33
  projects, 5–6
computer-supported collaborative learning (CSCL), 7, 112
  emergence of, 8
computer-supported collaborative work (CSCW), 112
Con-ciencia project, 93
conduct. *See* choice of conduct
confidence, 11, 12, 142
  in ACT, 166
  competence and, 84
  definition of, 83–84
  expression of, 84
  in TangibleK program, 142
  Zora virtual world and, 157
conflict, development and, 22
connection, 6, 11, 12, 104
  in ACT, 167
  in TangibleK program, 143
  in Zora virtual world, 157
consequences, 94
Constructionism, 6, 62, 136
  concept of, 7
  on content creation, perspective of, 68
  definition of, 14

educational technology and authoring environments of, 7
  learning environments of, 38–39
  Papert on, 14
  PTD and, 15
  software, 25, 83
  tools of, 7–8, 14
Constructivism, 14
consumption, production and, 37–38, 40, 42, 64, 67
contact, with participants, 138
  in ACT, 172
  in TangibleK program, 153
  in Zora virtual world, 164
content creation, 11–12
  in ACT, 166
  competence increase and, 67–68, 141
  Constructionist perspective on, 68
  TangibleK program, 141
  in Zora virtual world, 156
context, of institution, 139
  in ACT, 173–74
  in TangibleK program, 155–56
  in Zora virtual world, 165
context, of practice, 13
contribution, 11, 12, 119–23, 155, 157
COPPA. *See* Children's Online Privacy Protection Act
Creative Hybrid Environment for Robotic Programming (CHERP), 28, 71–72, 72f, 85, 116–17, 150
  download process, 151f, 152
creative process, 82–83
creativity, 12, 24, 82–85
  in ACT, 166
  computers and, 83
  discipline and, 83
  for problem solving, 82
  spiraling creative cycle of, 84–85
  in TangibleK program, 141–42
  in Zora virtual world, 156–57
Crouser, Jordan, 71, 124–26
CSCL. *See* computer-supported collaborative learning
CSCW. *See* computer-supported collaborative work
culture, 77, 97–98
curriculum, 134–39
  of ACT, 169, 170t–171t
  of TangibleK program, 147t–150t
  of Zora virtual world, 160, 161t

cyberbullying, 104, 105
cybernetics, 101–2

decision-making
  moral, 42, 91, 93
  political, 42
democracy, 77, 120
design. *See also* digital design
  of ACT, 168–74
  Brown on, 64
  children and, 64–65
  contextual factors of, 3
  definition of, 63–64
  development and, 4
  digital, 3, 63–64
  education, 39
  knowledge as, 39
  landscape, 3–4
  learning through, 38
  principles of, 64
  of toys, 24
  of Zora virtual world, 159–65
desires, 43
development. *See also* Positive Technological Development
  adolescent, 16–17, 46, 52
  of children, 3–5
  of competence, 36–37
  of computational thinking, 68–69
  conflict and, 22
  design and, 4
  eight stages of, 21–22
  identity and, 44, 46–47, 160
  milestones of, 21–22, 137, 146–47, 160, 169
  of morals, consequence and, 94
  of morals, six stages of, 92
  positive youth, 15–18
  PTD model trajectory of personal, 13*f*
  social interaction, 42
  technology and, 23, 34, 64
developmental milestones
  of ACT, 169
  of Zora virtual world, 160
deviantART, 107–8
DevTech, 28, 71, 112
digital art, 77–78
digital design, 3, 63–64
digital literacy, 76
digital manipulatives, 29
Digital Mom, 105

discipline, creativity and, 83
diSessa, Andy, 70
diversity, 138
  of ACT, 171–72
  of TangibleK program, 152
  of Zora virtual world, 163
DJ-ing, 87–88
doubt, 22, 23, 28
Druin, Allison, 65
Durrell, Lawrence, 3

"The Easiest Way to Jailbreak ANY Firmware iPhone!", 57
education
  design, 39
  entertainment and, 83
  principles of, 33
educational software, 7, 23–24, 83
educational technology
  CAI, 7
  Constructionist authoring environments and, 7
  CSCL, 7, 8
  ITS, 7
edutainment, 83
egocentrism, 160
Eliot Pearson Department of Child Development (Tufts University), 6
e-mail, 104
Emilia, Reggio, 144
empathy, 64
engineering, 78–79
engineering licenses, 141, 142*f*
entertainment, education and, 83
Entertainment Software Association (ESA), 40
epistemological pluralism, 38
Erikson, Erik, 21, 22, 36, 53, 146–47
ESA. *See* Entertainment Software Association
ethics, 95
Ettinger, Alyssa, 60–61, 105–6
EverQuest, 121
experience
  knowledge-based models of, 136
  praxis-based models of, 136
  ten dimensions of positive youth, 137–39

Facebook, 56, 57, 99, 104, 115–16, 126–27
The Facebook Safety Center, 105

failure, 87
family dynamics, 50
fan fiction, 98
fidelity, 53, 169
filtering, software, 134
Fisher-Price Smart Cycle, 27
Flannery, Louise, 31–32
football, 50–51
freedom, 91
friendship, 116–18
frustration, 142

G4C. *See* Games for Change
Gaia, 55
games, 26, 95. *See also specific types*
  community and, 59–60
  computer, 23, 35, 59–60
  definition of, 40
  MMORPG, 59
  video, 40–42, 50–51, 59–60, 96–97, 120–21
  web-based simulation, 72
Games for Change (G4C), 120–21
gender, 124–26
Gilligan, Carol, 92
global community, 60–61
goals, 70
Gogel, Hannah, 126–27
GoodPlay Project, 95
The Good Teen (Lerner), 16–17, 113
Google Analytics, 61
Grand Theft Auto, 97
guilt *vs.* initiative, 22, 147

Habbo world, 54, 55
hacking, 57
Heschel, Abraham Joshua, 52, 54
"Hide and Seek With Koko," 35
high school students, video games and, 96–97
Hillel, 119
Holocaust, 47–48
Horn, Mike, 71
HTML, 80–81
human capacity, technology and expansion of, 87–88
human-computer interfaces, 65

Iassogna, Jennifer, 26
identity, 67
  civic, 131–32
  community and, 53

development and, 44, 46–47, 160
exploration of, 52, 54–55
formation, 21
human, 5
moral, 93
religion and, 46–48
role confusion *vs.*, 52–53, 169
technology and formation of, 54
wireless hangouts and, 56
IDEO, 64
imagination, 24, 85
immersion, 136–37
improvement, of skills, 84
income, social networks as source of, 56–58
individual, society and, 119
individuality, 53
Industrial Revolution, 16
industry *vs.* inferiority, 36, 44, 64, 67
information, Internet and, 55
Information Age, 40
Information and Communication Technology Standards, 9
initiative *vs.* guilt, 22, 147
insecurity, 135
Instructionism, 136
integrity, 168
intelligent tutoring systems (ITS), 7
Internet, 8, 26, 39, 43, 80–81
  civic engagement through, 42, 119–23, 169
  communication, 102–3
  on culture, impact of, 77
  information and, 55
  safety, 104–5
  saving lives with, 123–24
  social capital, 102–3
interpersonal assets, 11
interpretation, communication and, 102
intrapersonal assets, 11
iPad, 30–31
iPhone, 57
isolation, 59–60
ITS. *See* intelligent tutoring systems

Jenkins, Henry, 78
Josephson Institute's Center for Youth Ethics, 93
journals, 141, 154
Judaism, 46–48, 52, 54
JumpStart 3D Virtual World, 24–25

Kaiser Family Foundation, 40–41
Kaiser Report, 40–41
Kay, Alan, 142
Kazakoff, Elizabeth R., 30–31
Kendall, Amber, 96–97
Kid Pix, 24, 25, 85
Kiger, David, 71
Kim, Jeewon, 97–98, 113–16, 123–24
kindergarten, 22, 94–95
knowledge as design, 39
knowledge-based models, of experience, 136
Kohlberg, Lawrence, 92
Koschman, Timothy, 7

landscape design, 3–4
landscapes, 3
language, 21, 27
Lanster, Lauren, 58–60
laws, for virtual worlds, 93–94
learning, 26, 112
   environments, Constructionist, 38–39
   objectives of TangibleK program, 149t–150t
learning by designing, 38
Lee, Brandon, 107–8
Lee, Kenneth Tae-Han, 87–88
Legend of Zelda, 98
LEGOS, 28, 31–32, 105–6, 142
   MINDSTORMS, 14, 79, 152
   robot, 116–18
Lerner, Richard, 15, 16–17, 84, 104, 113, 119
letters, 29
Lifelong Kindergarten, 15
Lisp, 14
LiveJournal, 113–15
Logo programming language, 7, 14, 15, 39, 69, 70, 71f
loyalty, values and, 53
Lucasfilm, 107

malls, 37, 43
manga, 97–98
manipulatives, 29
Matas, Jared, 116–18
McLuhan, Marshall, 102
media literacy, 76
Medieval periods, 16
medium, of communication, 102
mentoring model, 137–38
   of ACT, 171
   of TangibleK program, 152

of Zora virtual world, 163
Merrill Lynch, 26, 33
Mi Ani Project, 93
microphone headset, 96
Microsoft Virtual Worlds, 161–62
Mindstorms: Children, Computers, and Powerful Ideas (Papert), 14
MMORPG. *See* multi-player online role-playing game
money, 47
morals
   consequence and development of, 94
   decision-making, 42, 91, 93
   development, six stages of, 92
   identity, 93
   judgment of children, 92
   reasoning ability, 92
Moses, 89
Moss, Ty, 56–58
motor skills, 21, 22, 25, 27
multimedia parks, 45–46
multi-player online role-playing game (MMORPG), 59
music, 87–88

The National Center for Missing and Exploited Children, 105, 134
National Robotics Challenge, 142–43
National Science Foundation, 28
needs, 43
Neopets, 43
NetSmartz.org, 105
Nintendo, 96, 98
Nintendo Wii, 50, 96, 105–6
No Preschooler Left Behind, 166
numbers, 29
NXT bricks, 79

objects, 27
online forums, 98
Otaku club, 97–98

Panwapa, 25–26, 33–35, 103
Panwapa Islander Cards, 34
Panwapa Kids Cards, 34
"Panwapa Movie Play-Along," 35
Papert, Seymour, 6, 8, 15, 38, 44
   on Constructionism, 14
   on technocentrism, 135
parents, 17
parks, 36–38, 44

The Partnership for 21st Century Skills, 39–40
patterns, 6
pediatric patients, virtual worlds for, 156–65
peers, 42, 103
personality, 87
Pew Internet and American Life Project, 41, 55, 121
photos, 104
Piaget, Jean, 14, 68, 92, 135
piano, 37–38
play, 22, 95
   computers and, 33
   patterns of, 24
playgrounds, 4, 24
   autonomy and, 22–23
   communication and, 103
   risks of, 22–23
   robots and, 28–29
   in suburban areas, 25
   virtual, 25–26, 33–35
playpens, 23
   communication and, 103–4
   Fisher Price Smart Cycle as, 27
   risks of, 23
policy, 133–34
political decision-making, 42
popular culture, 77
portfolios, 154
Positive Technological Development (PTD), 4, 5, 56. *See also* choice of conduct; collaboration; communication; community building; competence; confidence; content creation; creativity
   ACT and framework of, 169*f*
   assets, 10–12, 13*f*, 17–18
   beginning of, 6
   behaviors, 11–12, 13*f*, 17–18
   case studies of, 140–74
   components of, 10
   Constructionism and, 15
   definition of, 7
   framework of, 62, 129*f*, 145, 146*f*, 158*f*, 159, 169*f*, 175
   goal of, 9, 10
   need for, 7–10
   personal development trajectory using, 13*f*
   TangibleK program and framework of, 146*f*
   theoretical model of, 10–12, 13*f*
   Zora virtual world and framework of, 158*f*, 159
positive youth development (PYD)
   assets, 15–18
   positive youth experience, 137–39
   technology and, 17
positive youth experience, 137–39
powerful ideas, of TangibleK program, 147*t*–148*t*
praxis-based models, of experience, 136
preadolescents, 160
preschool, 22
privacy, 99–100, 104, 105, 133–34
problem solving, 23, 64, 82
production, consumption and, 37–38, 40, 42, 64, 67
programming
   3-D, 73, 162
   AgentSheets, 72–73
   Alice, 73
   Cascading Style Sheets, 81
   CHERP, 28, 71–72, 72*f*, 85, 116–17, 150, 151*f*, 152
   environments, 39, 40, 68
   HTML, 80–81
   Logo language of, 7, 14, 15, 39, 69, 70, 71*f*
   SAGE, 73*f*, 74–76, 93
   Scratch, 15, 39, 48–49, 71*f*, 89–90
   tangible, 27–28
   Tern, 71
   virtual blocks, 71–72
   virtual worlds, 73
program scale, 138
   of ACT, 172
   of TangibleK program, 152–53
   of Zora virtual world, 163–64
Project for Awesome, 58
psychology. *See* applied developmental psychology
PTD. *See* Positive Technological Development
purpose, 53
PYD. *See* positive youth development

Quest Atlantis, 95, 121

Rare Animal Cards, 34
relationships, virtual worlds and, 121–22

religion
    identity and, 46–48
    Judaism, 46–48, 52, 54
Renaissance, 82
Repenning, Alex, 72
Resnick, Mitchel, 6, 15, 37–38, 83
responsibility, 91
risks
    COPPA, 133–34
    of playgrounds, 22–23
    of playpens, 23
    of virtual worlds, 103–4
robots, 15, 32, 65, 78–79, 93, 145. See also
        Creative Hybrid Environment for
        Robotic Programming
    LEGO, 116–18
    playgrounds and, 28–29
    robotic kits, 27–29
    SAGE, 73f, 74–76, 93
    TangibleK program, 94–95,
        140–56
role confusion, identity vs., 52–53, 169
role models, 93
routine, 146
rules, 146
Rwanda, 126–27

Sabbath, 52, 54–55
safety, 25
    COPPA, 133–34
    Internet, 104–5
SAGE. See Storytelling Agent Generation
        Environment
Sandvi, Ashley, 50–51
Sawyer, Keith, 82
"Schindler's List," 47
Scratch programming language, 15, 39,
        48–49, 71f, 89–90
The Search Institute, 10
The Second Half (Turkle), 176
Second Life, 55, 162
self-efficacy, 84
self-esteem, 67
self-expression, 8
self-monitoring, 70
self-organization, 93–94
self-reflection, 56
Selman, Robert, 92
Sesame Workshop, 26, 33–34
shame, 22, 23, 28
Shannon, Claude, 101

siblings, 109–10
SimCity, 121
The Sims, 85–87
six C's. See choice of conduct;
        collaboration; communication;
        community building; content
        creation; creativity
skills, improvement of, 84
Skype, 104
smart toys, 176
social gaming, 42, 95
social interaction, 42
social media, 54, 76, 95. See also
        blogging
    connection through, 115–16
    Facebook, 56, 57, 99, 104, 115–16,
        126–27
    income with, 56–58
    LiveJournal, 113–15
    Skype, 104
    Tumblr, 60–61
    Twitter, 57
    YouTube, 56–58
social networking, 104
society, 91, 119
software, 111
    art, 77–78
    for autonomy, 67
    Constructionist, 25, 83
    development cycle, 69
    DJ-ing, 88
    educational, 7, 23–24, 83
    ESA, 40
    filtering, 134
    policy, 133–34
Sony PlayStation, 96
Sony PlayStation 2, 50
space, 3
spatial reasoning, 160
SpeedChat, 103
SpeedChat Plus, 103
Spielberg, Steven, 47
spiraling creative cycle, 84–85
sports, 50–51, 60–61
state of flow, 83
stereos, 37–38
StopCyberbullying.org, 105
Storytelling Agent Generation Environment
        (SAGE), 73f, 74–76, 93
Sullivan, Amanda, 99–100
symbols, communication and, 26

TakingITGlobal, 120
TangibleK program, 94–95, 112, 131
   access environment in, 155
   assessment of, 153–54
   case study, 140–56
   choice of conduct in, 144–45, 155
   collaboration in, 142, 143f, 155
   communication in, 143–44, 155
   community building in, 144, 155
   confidence in, 142
   connection in, 143
   contact with participants, 153
   content creation in, 141
   creativity in, 141–42
   curriculum of, 147t–150t
   developmental milestones of, 146–47
   diversity of, 152
   institutional context in, 155–56
   learning objectives of, 149t–150t
   mentoring model of, 152
   portfolios, 154
   powerful ideas of, 147t–148t
   PTD framework and, 146f
   robots, 94–95, 140–56
   rubric of levels of understanding in, 154t–155t
   scale of, 152–53
   technology of, 150–52
   video journals, 154
tangible languages, 27
tangible programming, 27–28
technocentric thinking, 135
technocentrism, 135
technological fluency, 9, 39–40
   concept of, 68–69
   definition of, 8
technological literacy, 39
   of children, 4, 5, 33
technology, 4, 5, 137
   of ACT, 170
   development and, 23, 34, 64
   educational, 7, 8
   human capacity expansion with, 87–88
   identity formation and, 54
   PYD and, 17
   of TangibleK program, 150–52
   viral marketing of, 56–58
   of Zora virtual world, 161–62
teens. See adolescence
The Ten Plagues, 89–90
Tern programming language, 71
terrible two's, 21
text messaging, 55
thinking
   computational, 68–69
   moral development and, 92
   technocentric, 135
   thinking about, 136
third places, 95
time management, 36
toddlers, 21
tolerance, 168
Toontown Online, 103
TopCode, 151
toys, 28
   computational powers of, 29
   design of, 24
   mess-proof, 27
   smart, 176
transgender community, 101–2
transmission model, of communication, 101–2
trust, 168
Tumblr, 60–61
Turkle, Sherry, 38, 44, 54, 176
Twitter, 57
typing, 24

values, 3, 15, 46, 53, 168, 176
video games, 40, 42, 50–51, 59–60, 120–21
   behavior and, 41
   high school students and, 96–97
video journals, 154
viral marketing, 56–58
virtual blocks (programming), 71–72
virtual community, 54, 109–10
virtual playgrounds, 25–26, 33–35
virtual reality, 3
virtual temple, 47
virtual worlds, 42–44, 103, 120
   government of, 93–94
   identity exploration and, 52, 54–55
   laws for, 93–94
   Microsoft Virtual Worlds, 161–62
   for pediatric patients, 156–65
   programming, 73
   risks of, 103–4
   social relationships and, 121–22
   Zora, 45–46, 46–48
vocabulary, 21
volunteerism, 169
voting, 120

Weaver, Warren, 101
Web site creation, 80–81, 124–26
"Wheels on the Bus," 30–31
Wiender, Norbert, 101–2
Wing, Jeannette, 68
wireless communication, 52
wireless hangouts, 54–56
word processing, 39
World Cards, 34
World of Warcraft, 56, 59, 96, 121

Xbox 360, 96
Xbox Live, 96, 97

YouTube, 56–58

Zora virtual world, 45–48, 93, 109–10, 121–22, 162*f*
   access environment of, 165
   ACT with, 166–74
   assessment of, 164
   choice of conduct in, 158

   collaboration in, 157
   communication in, 157
   community building in, 157–58
   competence through, 156
   confidence in, 157
   connection in, 157
   contact with participants in, 164
   content creation in, 156
   context of institution in, 165
   creativity in, 156–57
   curriculum of, 160, 161*t*
   design dimensions of, 159–65
   developmental milestones of, 160
   diversity of, 163
   inspiration and motivation for, 55–56
   laws for, 93–94
   mentoring model of, 163
   for pediatric patients, 156–65
   PTD framework and, 158*f*, 159
   purpose of, 131–32
   scale of, 163–64
   technology of, 161–62